BRAIDING

BRAIDING

Easy
Styles
for
Everyone

Diane Carol **Bailey**

Jamie Rines **Jones**

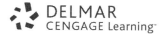
DELMAR
CENGAGE Learning

Australia • Brazil • Japan • Korea • Mexico • Singapore • Spain • United Kingdom • United States

PERSONAL CARE COLLECTION

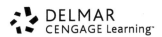

Braiding: Easy Styles for Everyone
Diane Carol Bailey, Jamie Rines Jones

Business Unit Director: Susan L. Simpfenderfer

Executive Editor: Marlene McHugh Pratt

Acquisitions Editor: Paul Drougas

Developmental Editor: Patricia A. Gillivan

Editorial Assistant: Rebecca McCarthy

Executive Marketing Manager: Donna J. Lewis

Channel Manager: Wendy E. Mapstone

Executive Production Manager:
    Wendy A. Troeger

For product information and technology assistance, contact us at
Cengage Learning Customer & Sales Support, 1-800-354-9706

For permission to use material from this text or product,
submit all requests online at **www.cengage.com/permissions**
Further permissions questions can be emailed to
permissionrequest@cengage.com

Library of Congress Control Number: 2001037237

ISBN-13: 978-0-7668-3764-5

ISBN-10: 0-7668-3764-5

Delmar
Executive Woods
5 Maxwell Drive
Clifton Park, NY 12065
USA

Cengage Learning is a leading provider of customized learning solutions with office locations around the globe, including Singapore, the United Kingdom, Australia, Mexico, Brazil, and Japan. Locate your local office at **international.cengage.com/region**

Cengage Learning products are represented in Canada by Nelson Education, Ltd.

For your lifelong learning solutions, visit **www.cengage.com/delmar**

Visit our corporate website at **www.cengage.com**

Notice to the Reader
Publisher does not warrant or guarantee any of the products described herein or perform any independent analysis in connection with any of the product information contained herein. Publisher does not assume, and expressly disclaims, any obligation to obtain and include information other than that provided to it by the manufacturer. The reader is expressly warned to consider and adopt all safety precautions that might be indicated by the activities described herein and to avoid all potential hazards. By following the instructions contained herein, the reader willingly assumes all risks in connection with such instructions. The publisher makes no representations or warranties of any kind, including but not limited to, the warranties of fitness for particular purpose or merchantability, nor are any such representations implied with respect to the material set forth herein, and the publisher takes no responsibility with respect to such material. The publisher shall not be liable for any special, consequential, or exemplary damages resulting, in whole or part, from the readers' use of, or reliance upon, this material.

Printed in the United States of America
4 5 6 7 11 10 09

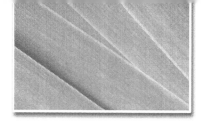

Contents

Working with Long Hair

SHAMPOOING AND BRUSHING

Shampooing and brushing long hair requires special techniques that not only make it easier for you but also cause less damage to long hair.

If you require a shampoo, use a gentle, all hair-type shampoo. With damaged or chemically treated hair, a moisturizing shampoo should be used, followed by a weekly, deep penetrating conditioner. There are several products available from professional haircare companies, and the choice is a matter of personal preference.

When shampooing your hair, apply shampoo to the scalp only, and then massage the entire scalp area using small circular motions. Now, rinse the hair while working the shampoo through to the ends. This is usually all that's required to cleanse the ends, since the primary goal is to clean the scalp without tangling the ends of the hair. Following this shampooing technique will cut down on the time needed for detangling and combing the hair.

Towel blot the hair by placing the towel over sections of the hair. Start at the top and squeeze as you work your way down. Do not rub. Rubbing will not remove excess water, but will instead create matting of the ends.

Change the towel whenever it gets too wet. Expect to use several towels.

At this point, a leave-in conditioner is strongly recommended. Use of this product will make combing the hair much easier. It also helps hold moisture in the hair when the hair is exposed to the heat of the sun, or the cold, drying weather of winter.

To comb long hair, start at the ends and gently work out the tangles while moving up one inch at a time. A large toothed, bone comb is effective in detangling the hair when it is wet. If the hair is clean and dry, a large paddle brush works well. Use the same technique of starting at the bottom and working up in 1" increments.

Now it's time to dry the hair. If you use a blowdryer, run your fingers through the hair from the scalp to the ends while you dry. Always go in the direction of the cuticle layer, not against it. If you need to save some time, sit under a hairdryer for about 5 minutes to remove excess water.

WET OR DRY?

If possible, it is best to work with dry hair. The only exception would be if you wanted a style that wasn't the best for your hair type. In this case, the hair requires dampening with water from a spray bottle, and the addition of gel or mousse, to hold the hair in place.

Working with dry hair means you don't have to walk around with wet hair. Also, as hair dries, it shrinks. If a braid is comfortable while the hair is wet, it will get tighter and uncomfortable as the hair dries. This could cause a headache.

Some people like to work with wet, gelled hair because it is easier to make it neat. This is true only if you have not perfected a hand position that stops the hair from sliding as you work with it. This hand technique will be discussed further in the book, and you will find that wet hair is no longer required to achieve neatness.

TOOLS OF THE TRADE

There are only 2 tools needed to work with long hair. They are:

1. A large 11" tail comb.
2. A square paddle brush.

The large tail comb in 11" long and is made of bone with 1/4" of space between the teeth. It is used for detangling wet hair and for back-combing dry hair. The tail portion of this comb is 6" long, which is required for making entire head sections. It is also long enough to hold all the hair at one time.

The square, anti-static, paddle brush is perfect for long hair for 3 reasons: First, these brushes usually have flexible rubber bristles. If you are brushing the hair and come to a knot, the tips of the bristles will bend and release the hair rather than ripping through the knot, which causes breakage. Second, the rubber bristles are seated in a padded base, which gives when pressure is applied. This adds to the assurance that the hair is not damaged or broken. And finally, removing hair from the brush is easier than with other brushes.

These are the only tools necessary when creating the long hair designs you'll find in this book. If you find other tools that work better for you, feel free to use them.

BACK-COMBING

Teasing with great vigor was the style at one time. It was achieved by using a teasing brush and brushing hard against the cuticle layer from the scalp to the ends. It resulted in very matted, tangled hair. This is not necessary with the styles you will be doing in this book. These styles use no teasing, but a few will require small amounts of back-combing.

Back-combing is done by placing a comb underneath a strand of hair. Starting very close to the base, roll the comb and apply medium pressure going against the cuticle layer. Usually, back-combing a strand once or twice is all that is needed to create the fullness required for these styles. Your goal is to make the strand you are back-combing fuller, and to prevent it from splitting or opening when you work with that strand.

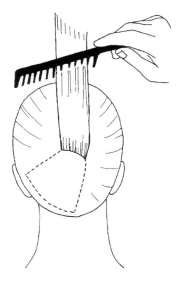

Remember, *back-combing should always be done with the hair combed in the direction in which you want the hair to go when finished.* Here is a common mistake seen in back-combing: Say the hair is in a ponytail at the crown, and you want to place a curl behind the left ear. People very often will back-comb the hair straight up, then try to force it behind the left ear. The result is usually buckling, or unevenness of that hair strand.

Now, take this same example with proper back-combing: Section out the hair you want placed behind the left ear, and then comb it in the direction in which you want the hair to lie. Next, back-comb this stand while keeping it in this position. Place your comb underneath and, starting very close to the base, back-comb the strand by rolling the comb while applying medium pressure. Smooth out the top if necessary, and then place the strand where you want it. If you are making a curl, there is no need to back-comb the ends, since they will be tucked under.

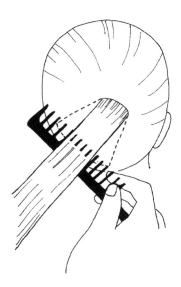

BOBBY PINS VS HAIRPINS

Bobby pins and hairpins look similar yet have a completely different purpose.

Bobby pins touch in the middle and are designed to hold weight. They are best suited when you need to anchor a weighted curl, or when you change the direction of the hair, such as in the bowtie (page 109) or the French twist with back-combing. For direction changes, make sure the tips cross each other. This gives them added strength in holding the hair where you want it.

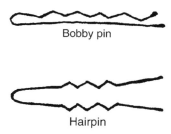

Bobby pin

Hairpin

Hairpins are used to help place hair that has already been secured with a bobby pin. For example, once a curl has been placed and secured where you want it, you might decide to spread the curl to make it wider. Spread the hair with your fingers, and then secure it with a hairpin to hold the strands in the new position.

A common question concerns the placement of pins in the hair. A basic rule is to pin exactly where your fingers are holding the hair. Very often, bobby pins are being inserted next to the fingers holding the hair. When you let go, the hair moves to the new pinned position. It takes a little practice, but it's worth it for perfect style placement every time.

The styles that follow in this book will offer examples for the use of bobby pins and hairpins. Suggestions will be made for the best pin to use.

THE PERFECT PONYTAIL

One of the most common problems people run into is getting the ponytail exactly where they want it while keeping the hair smooth. The main reason the hair doesn't stay smooth is because people try to tighten it after rubberband placement. Following are 2 different ways to make a ponytail without ever tightening it. Try both, and then decide which works best for you.

Ponytail #1

You will need 2 bobby pins and an elastic band (preferably fabric covered).

1. Attach 2 bobby pins to rubberband as shown.

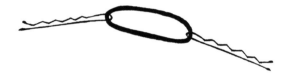

2. Put left hand where you want ponytail to be placed and brush hair into it. Holding hair securely, twist ponytail 1/4 turn clockwise.

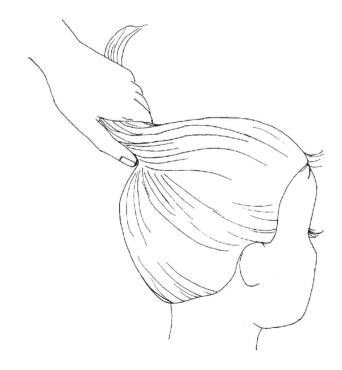

3. Insert one bobby pin into the top of the ponytail next to scalp. Hold securely with index finger. Allow other bobby pin to hang freely on the right side of ponytail.

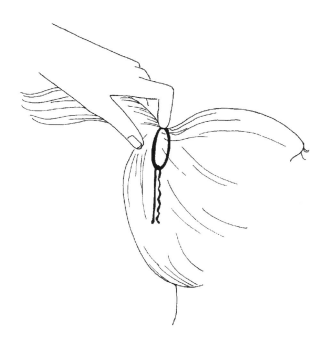

4. With right arm, reach over top of ponytail. With right hand, reach under ponytail to grab free-hanging bobby pin. Pull rubberband at least 1 1/2 times around ponytail.

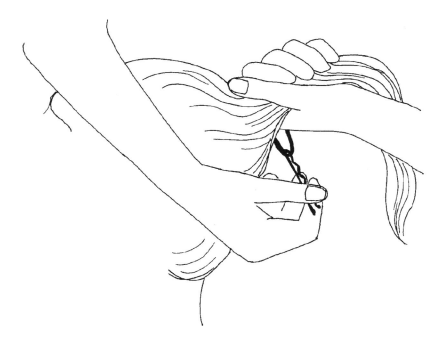

5. Insert free bobby pin into ponytail under the rubberband along the scalp.

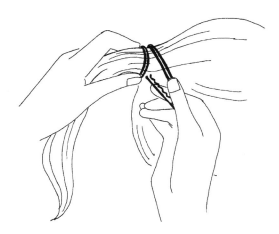

Ponytail #2

You will need 1 bobby pin and 1 rubberband (preferably fabric covered).

1. Attach bobby pin to rubberband as shown.

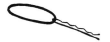

2. Put your left hand where you want the ponytail to be placed and brush hair into it. Hook the rubberband over your left thumb and allow the bobby pin to hang free.

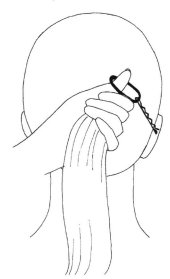

3. With your right hand, grab the free-hanging bobby pin and pull it underneath the ponytail, and then pull bobby pin through the rubberband.

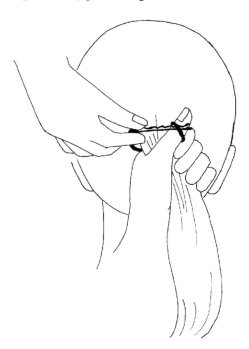

4. Pull the bobby pin back underneath the ponytail, and go back around the ponytail at least 1 time.

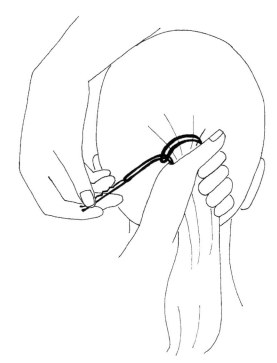

5. Insert free bobby pin into ponytail between the rubberband and scalp.

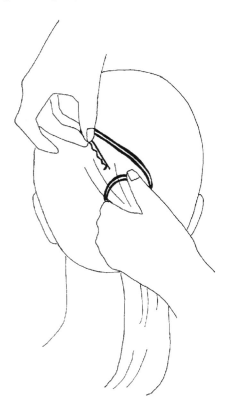

ACCESSORIES

Some of the following styles use ribbon to create the finished look. Here are some questions commonly asked about purchasing ribbon.

How wide should the ribbon be? The styles in this book use a ribbon no wider than 1/2". A personal favorite is 1/4" wide. It is easier to work with and it doesn't make the style quite as stiff.

What kind of ribbon is best? The ribbon should be as slick as possible. Metallic ribbons are fun, but they rarely have a smooth finish. When the ribbon is not smooth, it can pull on the hair and make the style look messy. The perfect test for ribbon is to run it over a silky fabric or panty hose and see if it catches. Once you have perfected using ribbons, you can successfully use ribbons that are not as slick, and still keep the style clean.

How long should the ribbon be? It is best to start with ribbon at least twice the length of the hair you are working on. Many of the styles don't require quite that much, but nothing could be worse than getting to the end of a style and finding out you need just a couple of inches more. Better safe than sorry, so cut the ribbon to twice the hair length to be sure.

Is there anything else besides ribbon that can be used? Yes, strings of pearls and strings of sequins can be used successfully. You can purchase these at most fabric or craft stores. They come on spools of 5 yards or more and can be cut to any length. But, again, you will not want to work with these 2 accessories until you have mastered using smooth ribbon. You will have a much better chance of a successful design.

While you are at the fabric or craft center, take time to look around. There are always treasures to be found and used in your hair designs. Some highly recommended items include the following.

Individual beads and pearls These are easily put onto a hairpin and placed in the finished design to dress it up. Colors recommended are gold, black, silver, and opaque white. Sizes recommended are from 2 to 4 mm. Following are directions for putting beads on hairpins and using them in your long hair designs.

1. Straighten a hairpin and slide bead onto it.

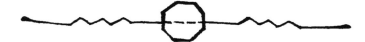

2. Bend the hairpin down firmly on either side of bead.

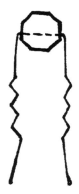

3. Bend one leg of the hairpin halfway up, as shown. This prevents the hairpin from slipping out when worn. Slide this accessorized pin into any hairstyle that needs to be dressed up for a special occasion.

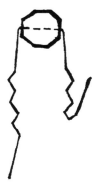

4. You can also tie bows or ribbons on the hairpin for a different look.

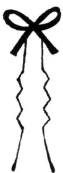

Easier still is to buy them already tied and just slip them onto a pin.

Silk flowers You can purchase tiny flowers wrapped in a small bundle. These are great to have on hand. Just cut them out of the bundle and insert them into the final design. If you use hairspray after you insert the flowers, it will help hold them in place. Real flowers, like baby's breath, are wonderful, too, but these are difficult to have on hand all the time.

Buttons Some of the buttons available today are tiny works of art. You can always hot glue or sew these onto a fabric-covered rubberband for a dressy or more fun look. Small rhinestone buttons can be added to a hairpin (follow directions for individual beads and pearls) for a stunning finish to an evening design.

Once you start looking around, you will become creative and come up with your own ideas. Belt buckles, tee-shirt clasps, and even gold charms have been used before, so don't be limited by the few things mentioned here.

CHAPTER 2

Long Hair Design

INTRODUCTION

This chapter takes you through a series of styles. It is designed so that you master one style before you proceed to the next. Each additional step is based on some technique learned in the style before it. Illustrations appear at every step to help you master the hand positions and technique of every style. Don't give up if it gets confusing. Start at step 1 again, and make your hands match the illustrations exactly. Keep practicing until the hand positions become comfortable before you move to the next style.

The following exciting styles are included in this chapter:

- Rope ponytail and chignon
- Rope braid
- Two-strand twist
- Two-strand twist with ribbon
- Two-strand ribbon braid
- Fishtail ponytail
- Fishtail
- French braid
- Dutch braid
- Twisting
- Knotting
- The bow
- The bowtie
- French twist

Rope Ponytail and Chignon

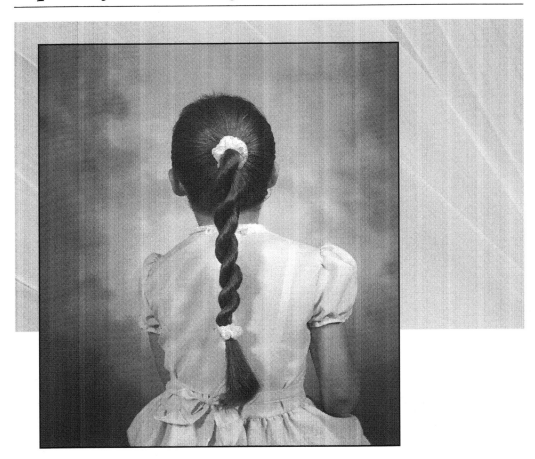

The rope ponytail is a true show stopper. The concept is simple, yet figuring out how to stop 2 twisted strands from coming unwound can be difficult. In order for 2 strands to stay twisted, they must go in opposing directions. Notice that the left-hand side is twisted to the right, yet the entire ponytail is twisted to the left.

This braid is best done on all one-length hair.

TIP! *The most common mistake made with this technique is twisting the left-hand side of the ponytail counterclockwise (or to the left). This will result in the twist's unwinding. If this happens, start over and make sure you twist the left-hand side of the ponytail clockwise (or to the right).*

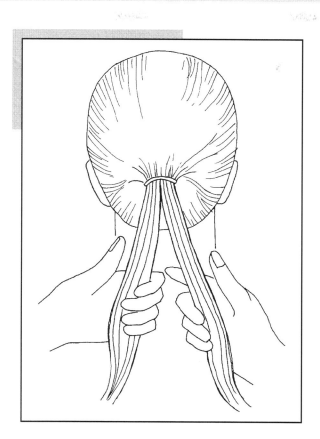

1. Begin with hair in ponytail.
Divide ponytail into 2 sections.

2. Twist left strand clockwise (to
the right) 2 or 3 times.

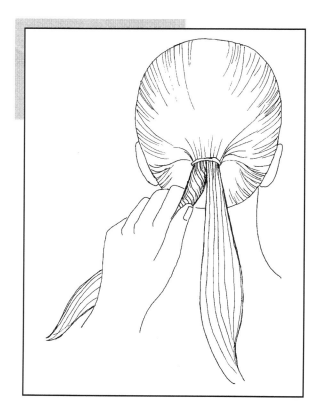

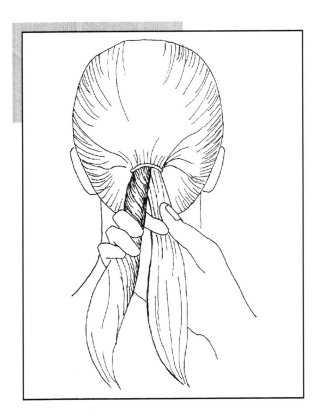

3. Place sections in your right
hand with index finger in between, hand palm up, as
shown.

4. Twist palm down (counterclockwise), right strand over left.

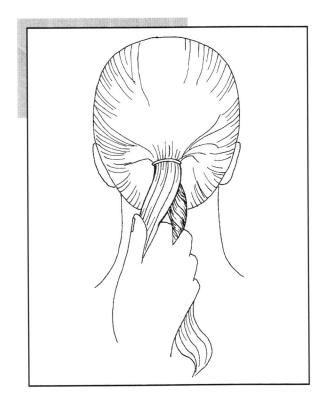

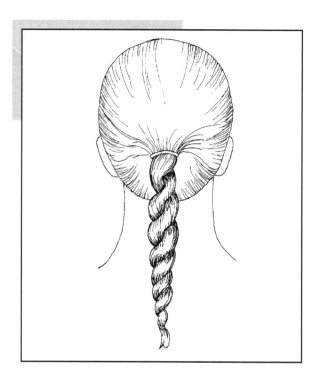

5. Repeat steps 2 through 4 until the ponytail is completely twisted. When this technique is done correctly, you can put a rubberband around the end of the ponytail and the ponytail will not come unwound.

6. Another option is to make a chignon from this rope. Begin twisting the rope ponytail counterclockwise around the rubberband.

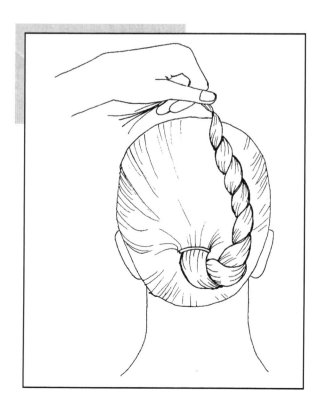

7. When you finish wrapping hair into a chignon, tuck ends under and secure with bobby pins.

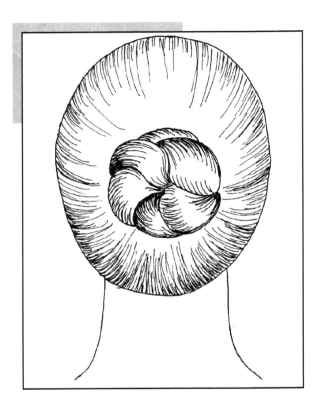

Rope Braid

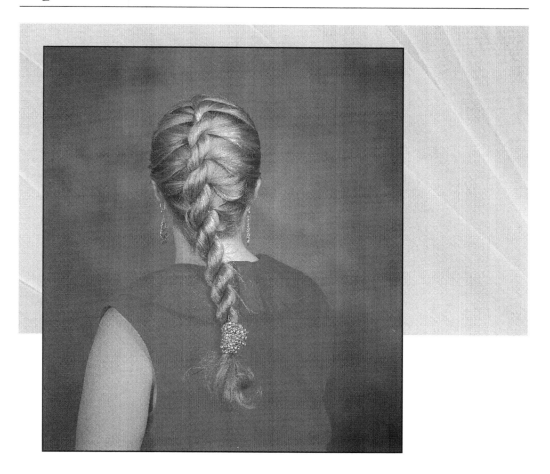

The rope braid is one of the most popular braids. It can be done on all one-length hair as well as long, layered hair.

TIP!	*You must add to both sides before you twist the right side over the left.*

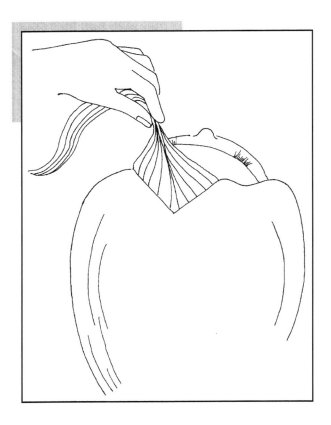

1. Take a triangle section of hair from the front. If there are bangs, begin behind them.

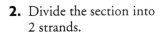

2. Divide the section into 2 strands.

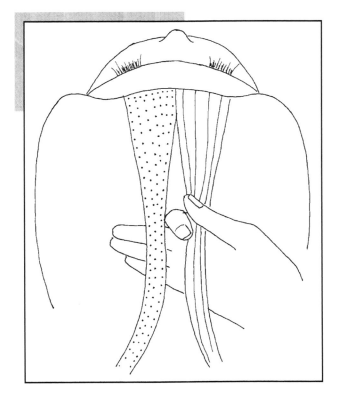

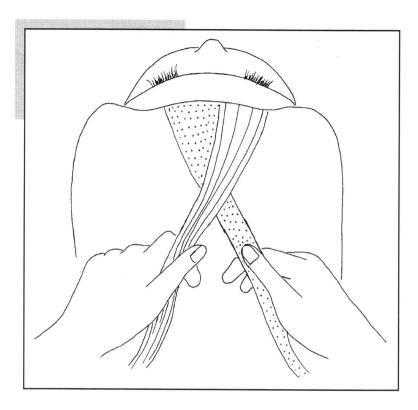

3. Cross the right strand over the left strand.

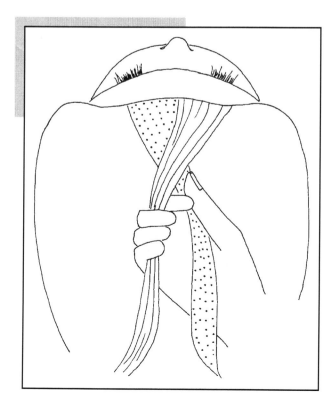

4. Place both strands in the right hand with the index finger in between, hand palm up, as shown.

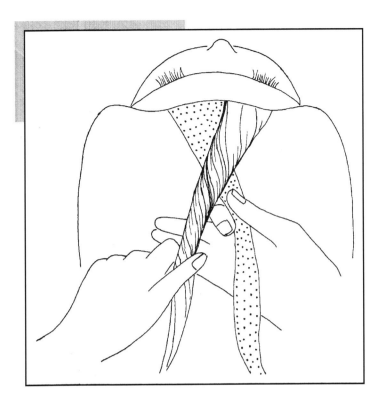

5. Twist the left strand 2 times clockwise, or toward the center.

6. Pick up a 1" section from the left side.

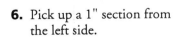
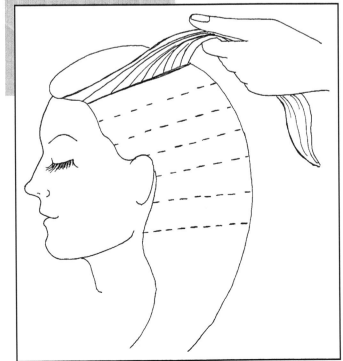

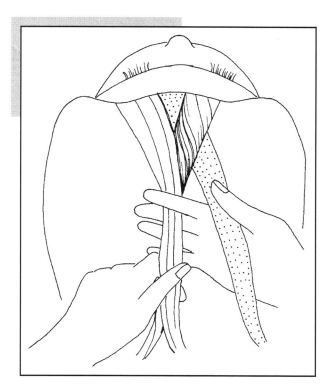

7. Add this section to the left strand.

8. Put both strands in the left hand with the index finger in between, hand palm up, as shown.

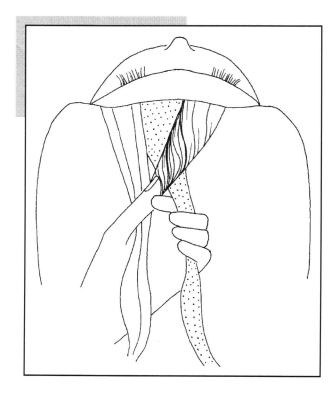

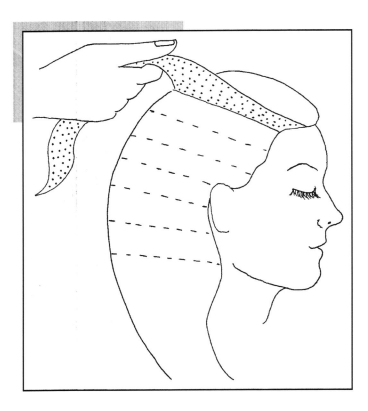

9. Pick up a 1" section from the right side.

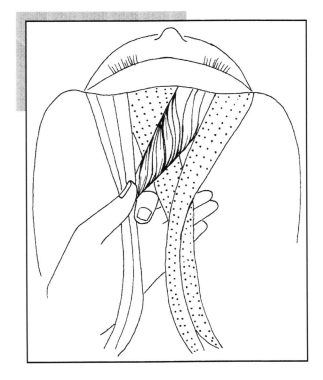

10. Add this section to the right side.

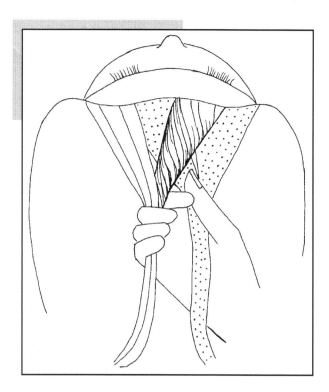

11. Put both strands in the right hand with the index finger in between, hand palm up, as shown.

12. With your hand in this position, twist toward the left (counterclockwise) until your palm is facing down.

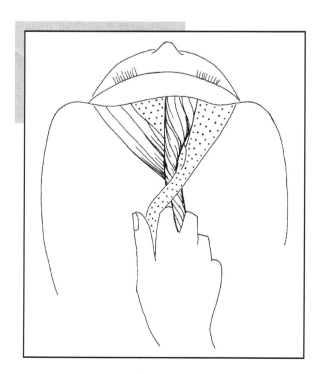

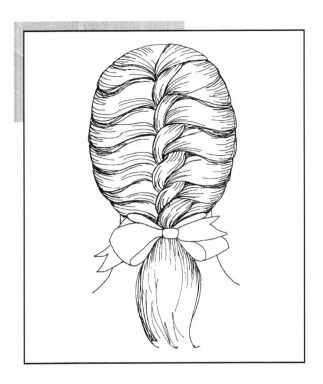

13. Repeat steps 4 through 11,
working toward the nape, until style is done. Use a rubberband to secure.

14. When you run out of sections
to pick up, you can repeat steps
2 through 4 of the rope ponytail. This will lock the braid
from coming unwound. Place a
rubberband around the ends
and let the ponytail hang free.

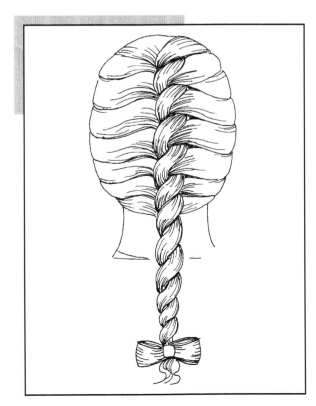

15. Another option would be to bobby pin the ends under in the nape area.

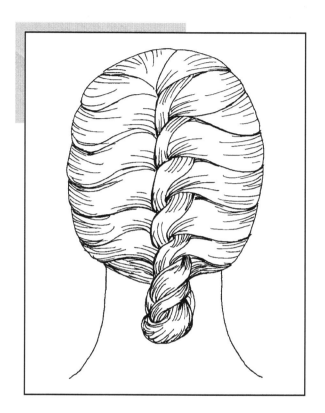

Two-Strand Twist

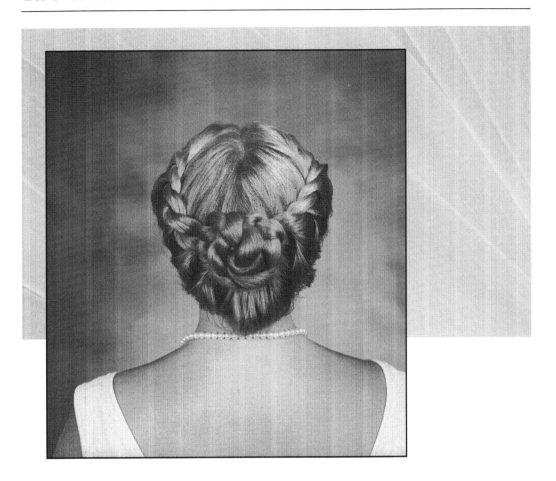

The 2-strand twist is another one of the most popular braids. It allows fullness on the sides and behind the ear and is perfect for the non-oval face. This style is done best on all one-length hair or hair that is shoulder length or longer.

TIP! *You must twist up toward the part. On the right side of the head, the right hand does the twisting toward the part, and, on the left side, the left hand does the work.*

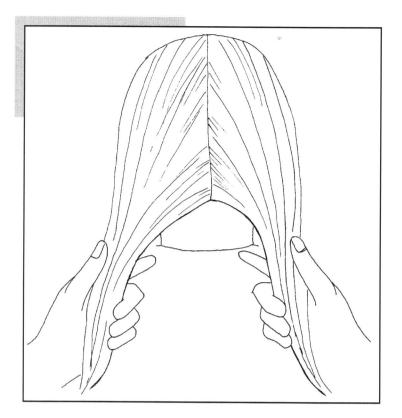

1. Divide hair into 2 sections.

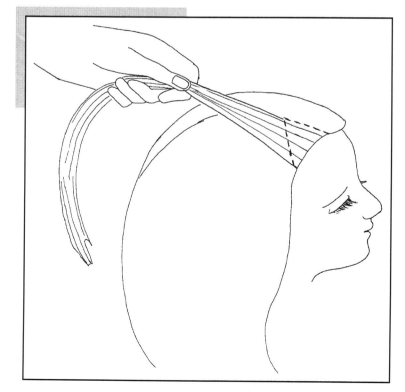

2. Starting on the right side, pick up a triangle section from the front.

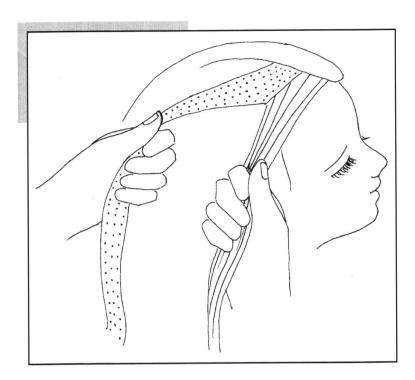

3. Divide this section into 2 strands.

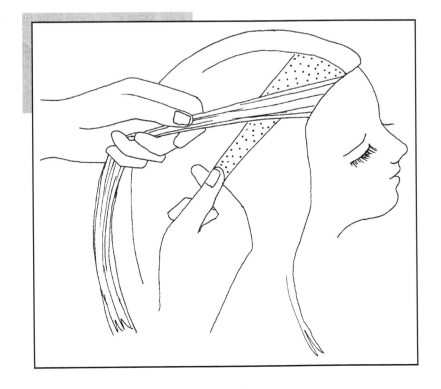

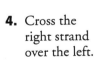

4. Cross the right strand over the left.

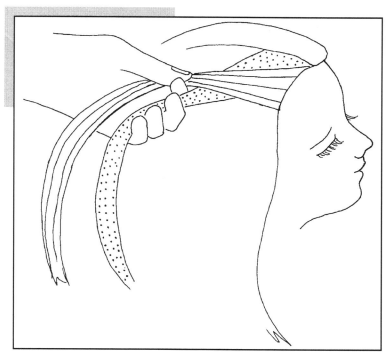

5. Place both strands in the left hand with the index finger in between. Keep the back of the left hand against the head at all times.

6. Starting at the hairline and continuing up toward your left hand, pick up a 1" section with your right hand.

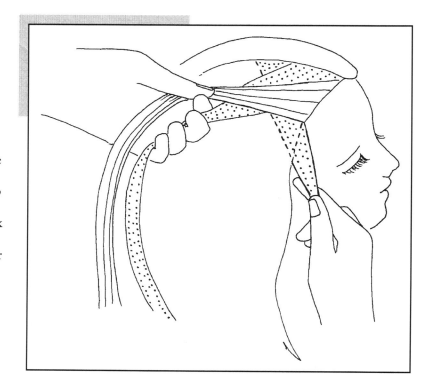

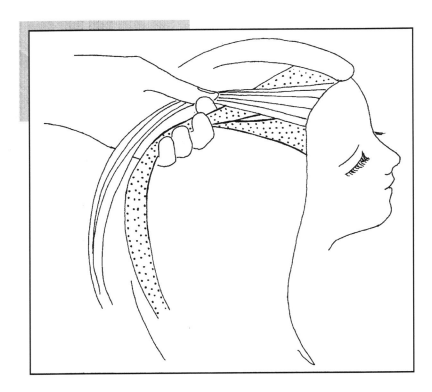

7. Add this section to the right (or bottom) strand.

8. Place these sections in your right hand, with the index finger in between.

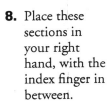
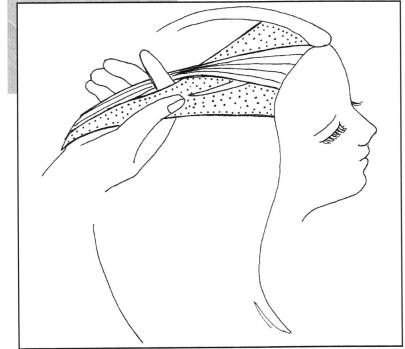

9. Twist right hand counterclockwise (the right strand twists over the left strand).

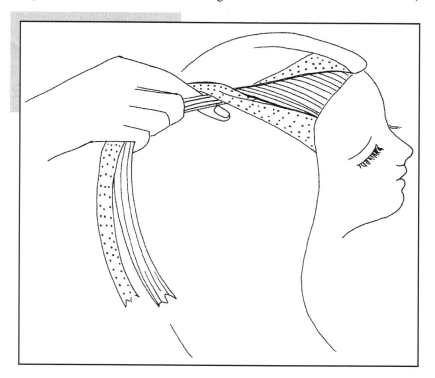

10. Repeat steps 5 through 9, picking up 1" sections of hair as you move down the head. Continue until you reach the nape and have no more hair to pick up. Clip this section out of your way.

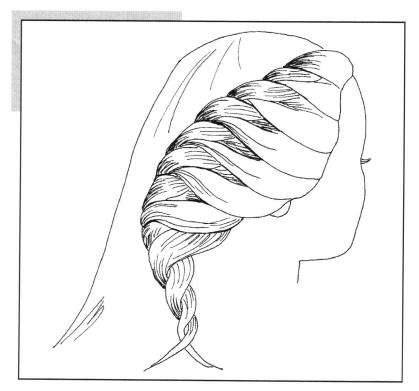

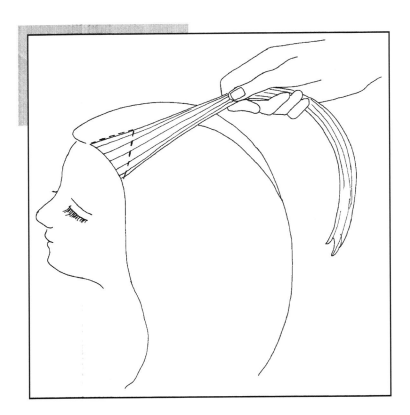

11. Starting on the
   left side, pick
   up a triangular
   section from
   the front.

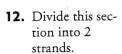

12. Divide this sec-
   tion into 2
   strands.

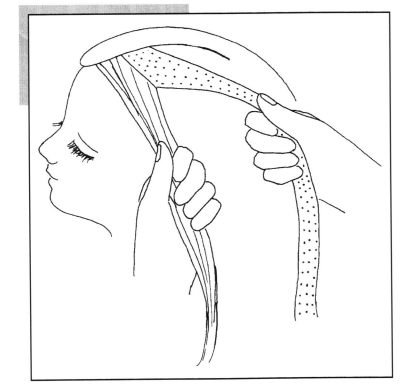

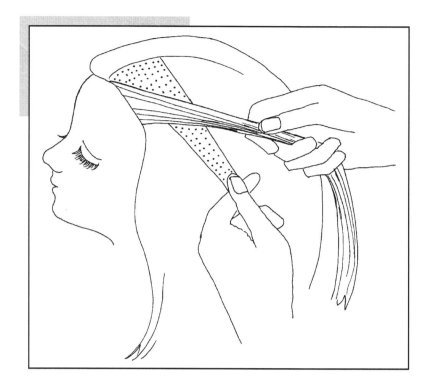

13. Cross the left strand over the right.

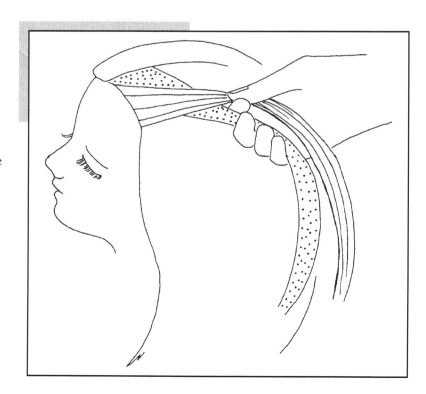

14. Place both strands in the right hand with the index finger in between. Keep the back of the right hand against the head at all times.

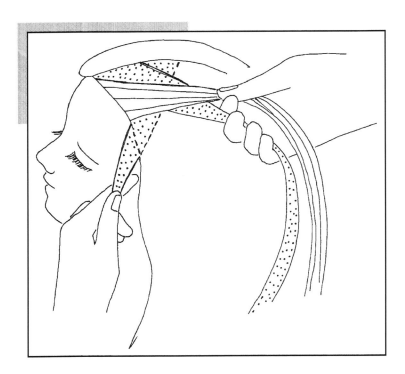

15. Starting at the hairline and continuing up toward your right hand, pick up a 1" section with your left hand.

16. Add this section to the left (or bottom) strand.

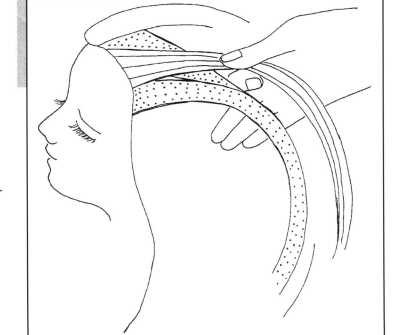

17. Place these sections in your left hand, index finger in between.

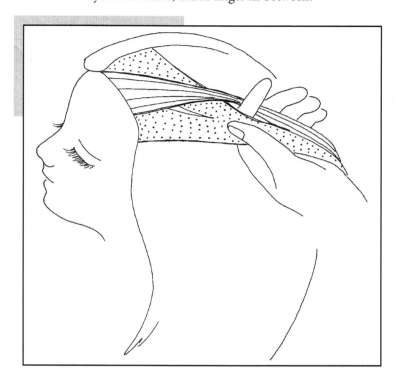

18. Twist left hand clockwise (the left strand twists over the right strand).

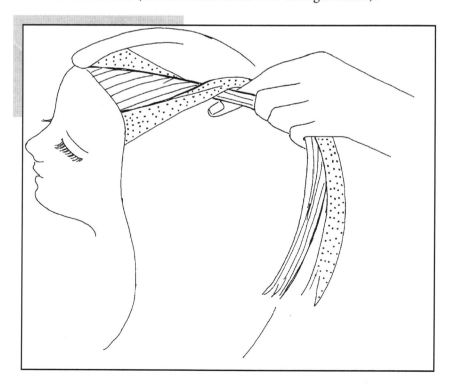

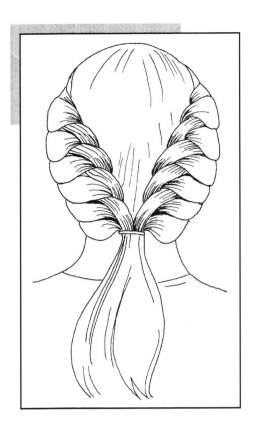

19. Repeat steps 14 through 18, picking up
1" sections of hair as you move down the
head. Continue until you reach the nape
and run out of hair. Bring both finished
sides together to form a ponytail. Secure
with a rubberband.

20. Another option would be to do the fishtail
ponytail. Cover the rubberband with hair,
make the ponytail, and then pin ends underneath. See the section on the fishtail
ponytail for more information.

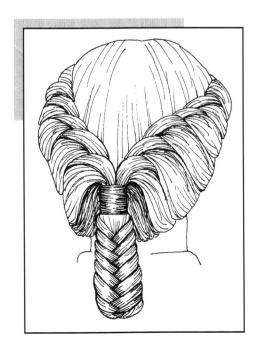

21. You could also leave the back down and do the 2-strand twist on the top portion of the head. This is a great option for all one-length, bob-line haircuts.

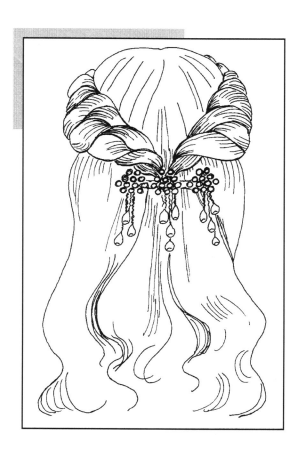

Two-Strand Twist with Ribbon

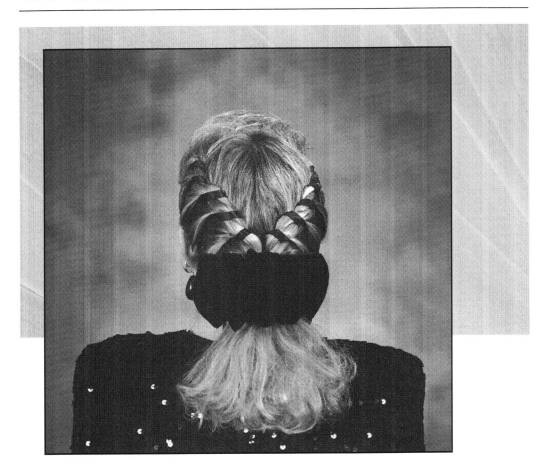

This is another beautiful way to dress up the 2-strand twist. Make sure you have perfected the 2-strand twist without ribbon before you attempt this version. It makes this style so much easier to master.

> **TIP!** *The ribbon never gets added to the hair strands. It is always passed after you twist the 2 hair strands over each other and before you pick up your next section.*

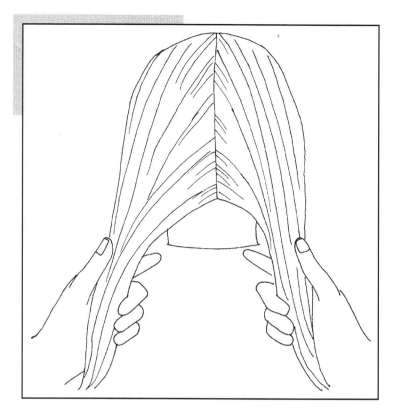

1. Divide hair into 2 sections as shown.

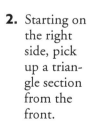 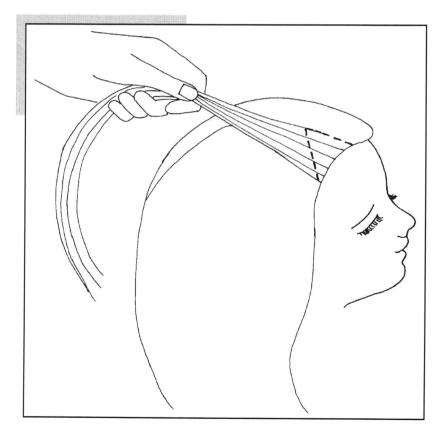

2. Starting on the right side, pick up a triangle section from the front.

3. Tie a ribbon to the inside of the triangle section. Push the ribbon toward the face and out of the way of the hair sections.

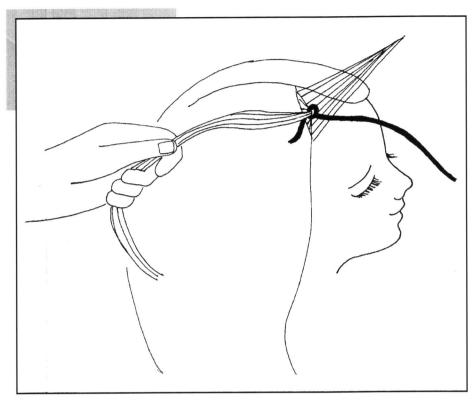

4. Divide the hair section into 2 strands.

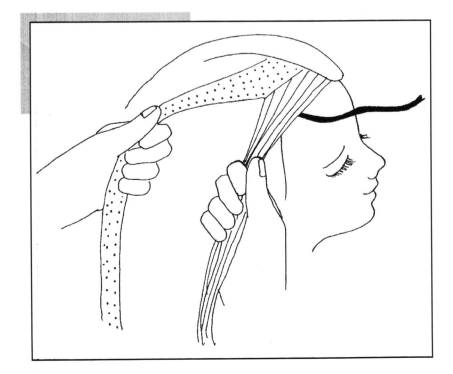

5. Cross the right strand over the left.

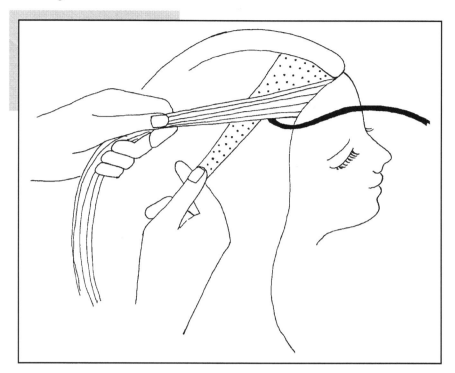

6. Place both strands in the left hand with the index finger in between. Keep the back of the left hand against the head at all times.

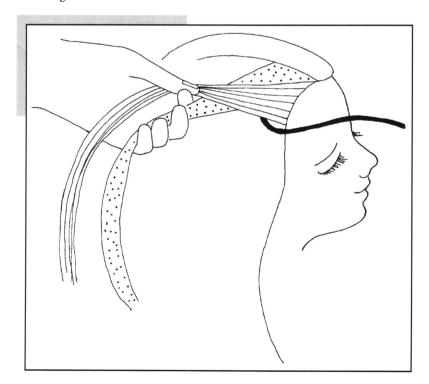

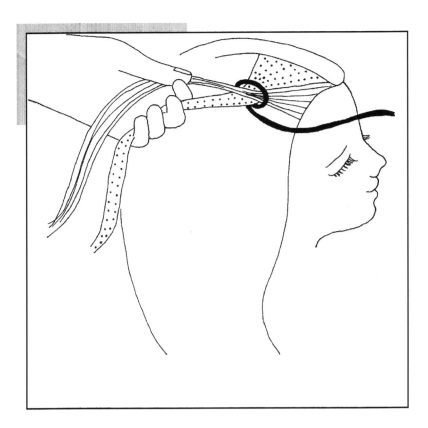

7. Now wrap ribbon counterclockwise completely around both sections. Push ribbon toward the face and out of the way of the hair section.

8. Starting at the hairline and continuing up toward your left hand, pick up a 1" section with your right hand.

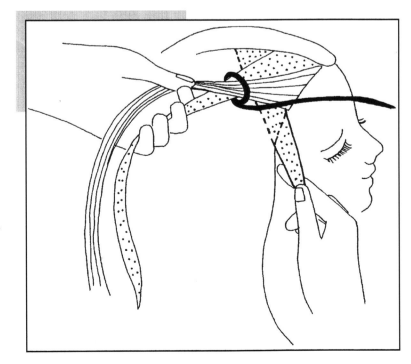

9. Add this section to the right (or bottom) strand.

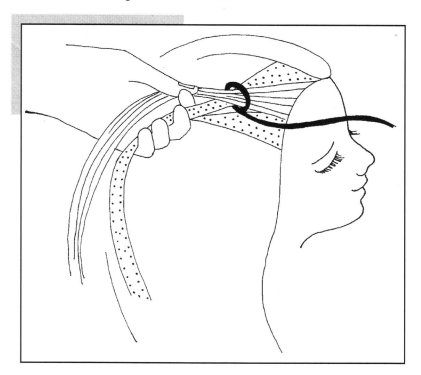

10. Place these sections in your right hand, with the index finger in between.

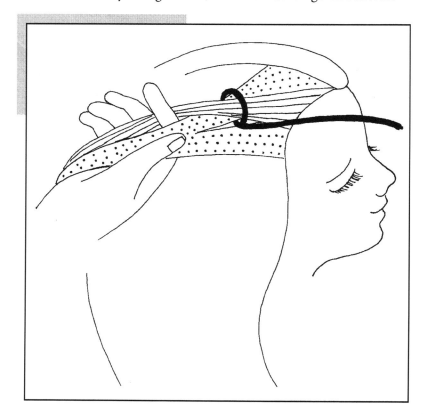

11. Twist right hand counterclockwise (the right strand twists over the left strand).

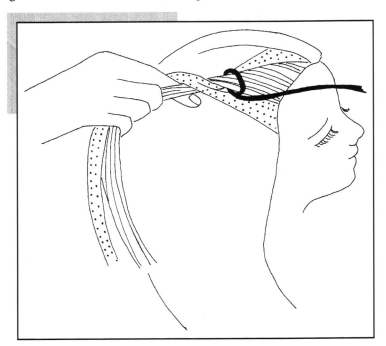

12. Repeat steps 6 through 11, picking up 1" sections of hair as you move down the head. Continue until you reach the nape and have no more hair to pick up.

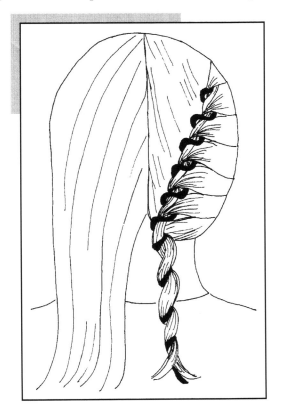

13. Starting on the left side, pick up a triangular section from the front.

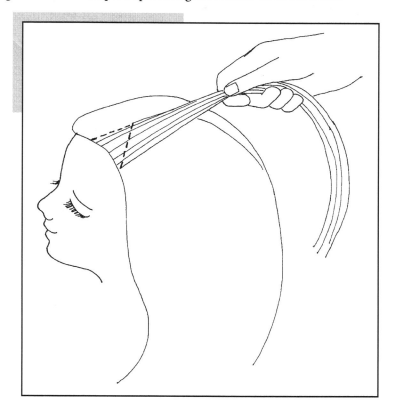

14. Tie a ribbon to the inside of the triangle section. Push ribbon toward the face and out of the way of the hair sections.

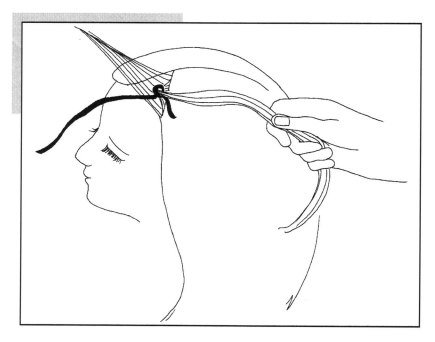

15. Divide the triangle section into 2 strands.

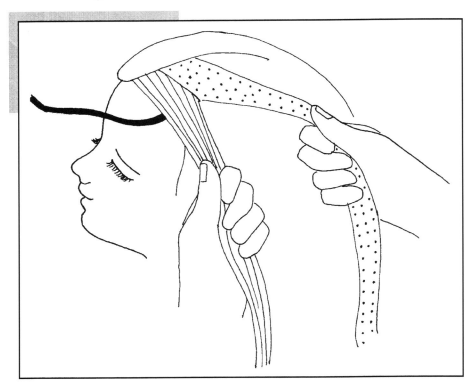

16. Cross the left strand over the right.

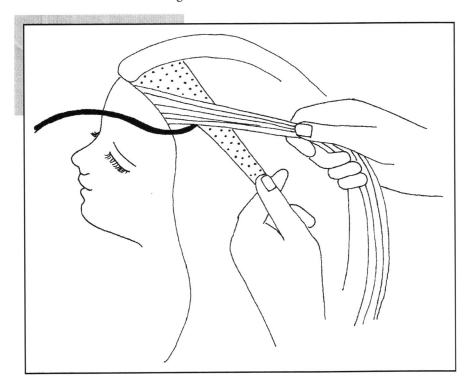

17. Place both strands in the right hand with the index finger in between. Keep the back of the right hand against the head at all times.

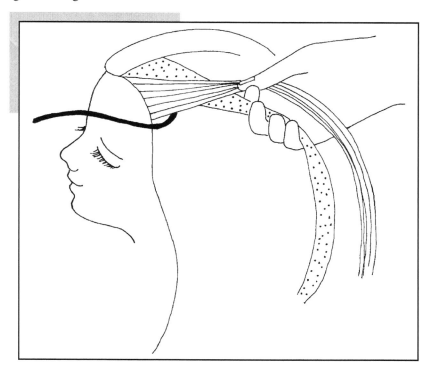

18. Wrap ribbon clockwise completely around both sections. Push ribbon forward and out of the way of the hair strands.

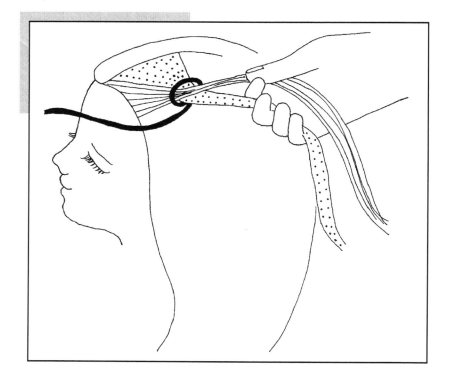

19. Starting at the hairline and continuing up toward your right hand, pick up a 1" section with your left hand.

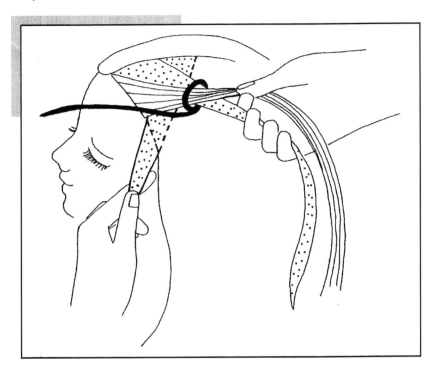

20. Add this section to the left (or bottom) strand.

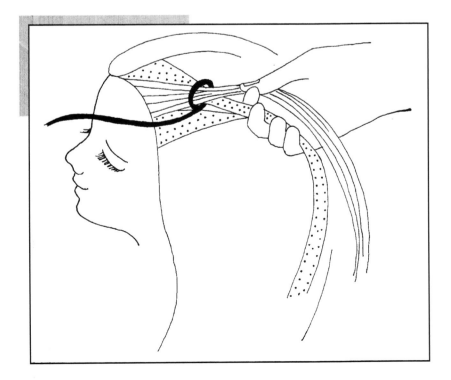

21. Place these sections in your left hand, index finger in between.

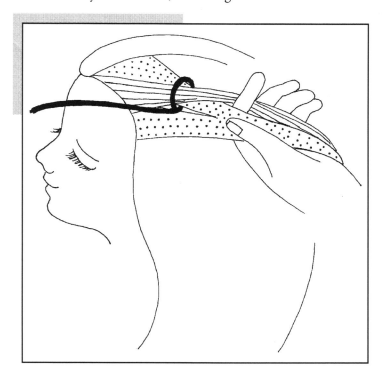

22. Twist left hand clockwise; left strand twists over the right strand.

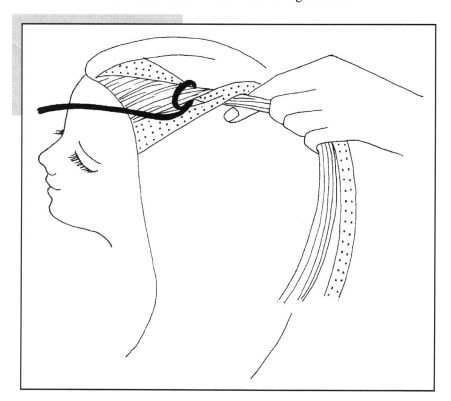

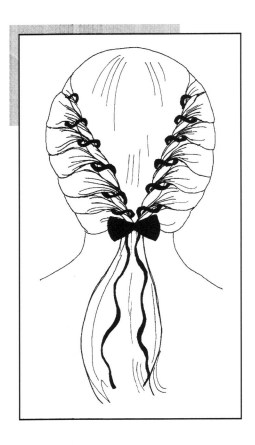

23. Repeat steps 17 through 22, picking up 1" sections of hair as you move down the head. Continue until you reach the nape and run out of hair. Bring the 2 finished sides together to form a ponytail.

24. Another option would be to wrap both ponytail sections with remaining ribbon, then wrap into a chignon.

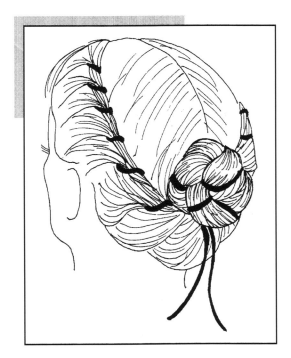

Two-Strand Ribbon Braid

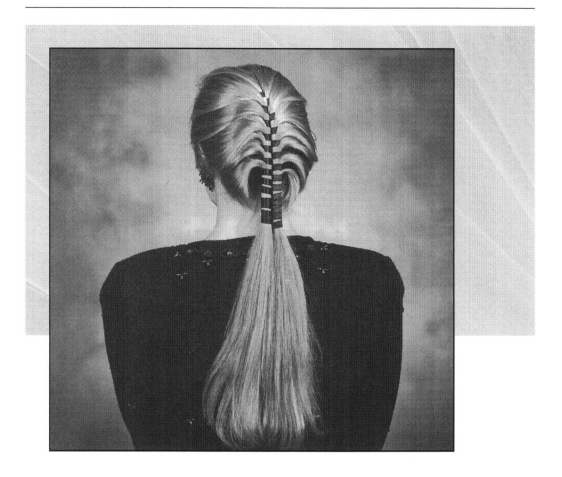

This is a perfect style for all one-length hair. It is popular for proms and weddings because ribbon that matches the dress can be braided into the hair. This style is also very easy to do.

> **TIP!** **The hair strands** never **twist or cross each other. The ribbon does all the work by making a figure 8 around the 2 strands.**

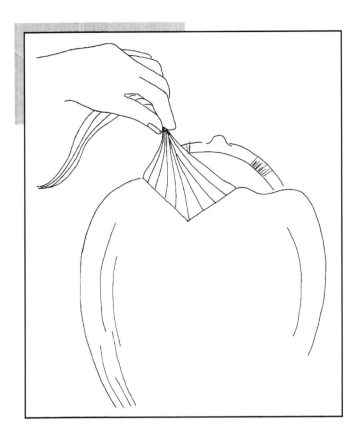

1. Take a triangle section of hair from the front. If there are bangs, begin behind them.

2. Divide the section into 2 strands. Tie a ribbon onto the left-side strand.

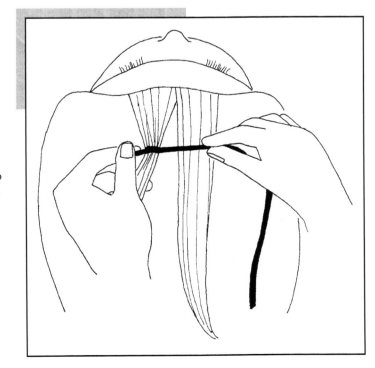

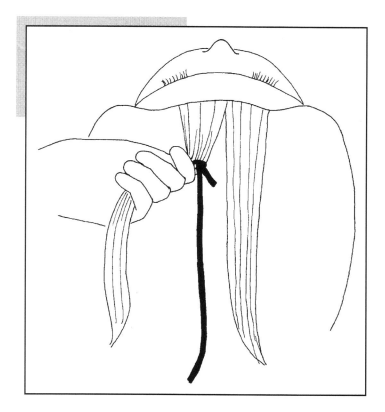

3. While holding the left-hand strand, drop the ribbon down to hang freely.

4. Pick up the right strand and place it in between the index and third fingers, hand palm up, as shown. Pick up the ribbon with your right hand and bring it under the right strand.

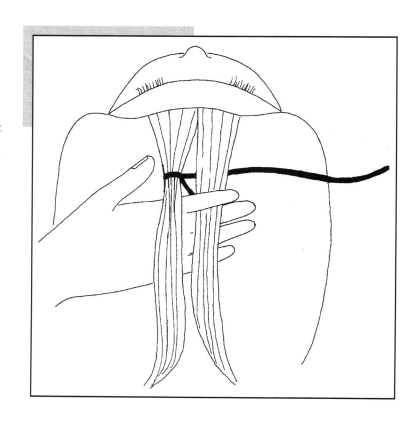

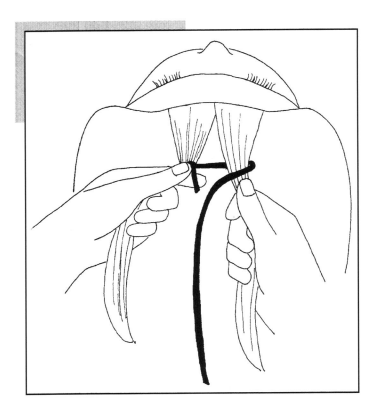

5. Then bring ribbon up and over the right strand. Drop the ribbon to let it hang freely between the 2 strands.

6. Place both strands in your right hand, index finger in between, hand palm up, as shown. Allow ribbon to hang freely.

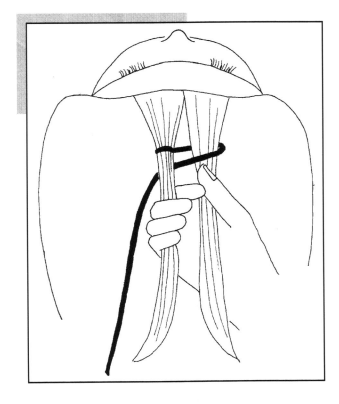

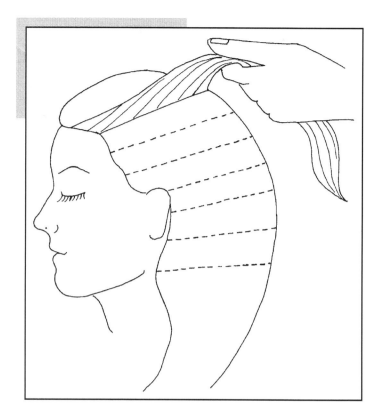

7. Pick up a 1" section on the left side.

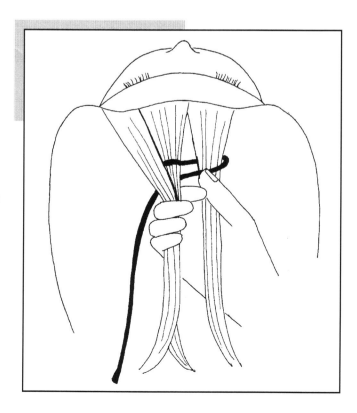

8. Add this section to the left strand you already have in your hand.

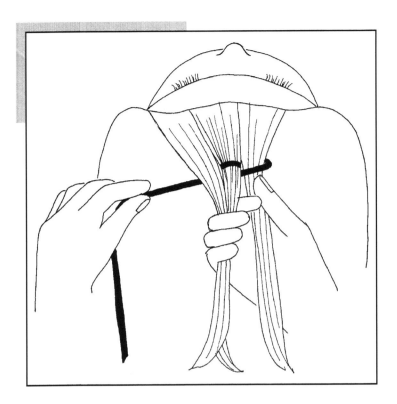

9. Pick up the ribbon with your left hand and bring it under the left strand.

10. Then bring ribbon up and over the left strand. Drop the ribbon to let it hang freely between the 2 strands.

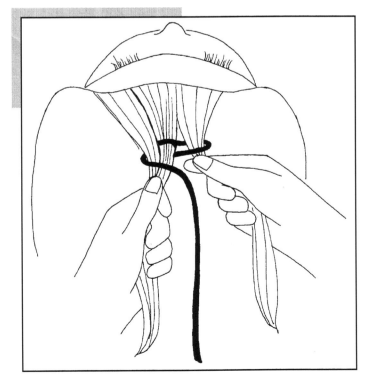
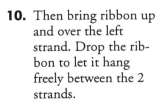

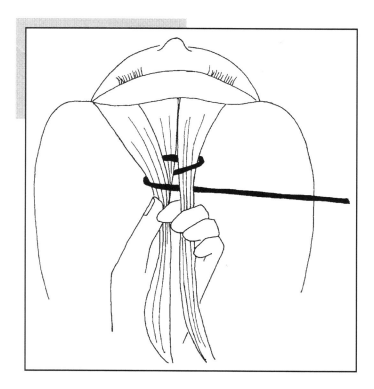

11. Place both strands in your left hand, index finger in between, hand palm up, as shown. Allow ribbon to hang free.

12. Pick up a 1" section on the right side.

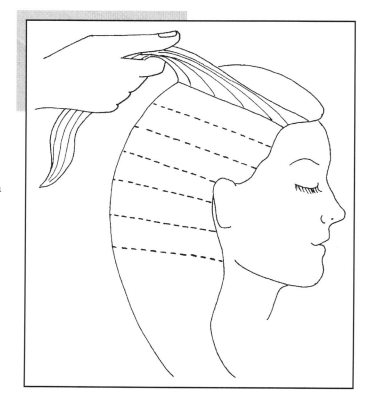

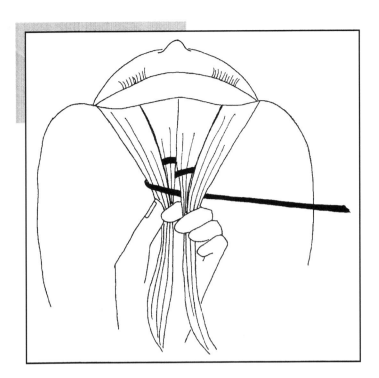

13. Add the section to the right-side strand already in your hand.

14. Pick up the ribbon with your right hand and bring it under, then up and over, the right strand. Allow ribbon to hang freely between the 2 strands.

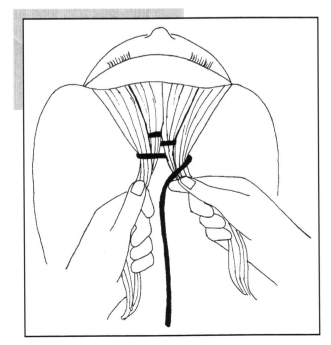

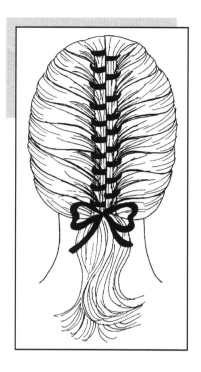

15. Repeat steps 6 through 14, moving down toward the nape with each 1" section picked up. When you run out of sections, secure braid with rubberband. Remainder of hair forms a ponytail.

16. Another option is to finish the ponytail by continuing to make a figure 8 with the ribbon to the ends of the hair.

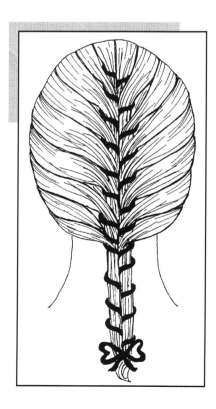

Fishtail Ponytail

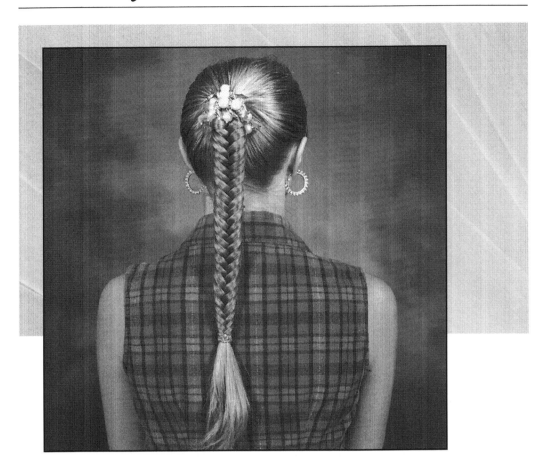

The fishtail is a very complicated-looking braid yet is actually one of the easiest braids to do. It is best done on dry, all one-length hair. It makes a very attractive ponytail by itself. It could also be a perfect way to finish off a ponytail combined with another type of braid such as the 2-strand twist.

 TIP! *When doing steps 2 and 4, make sure you reach behind the free-hanging section. If you take the sections from the top, they will not wrap around the sides and the finished look will be affected.*

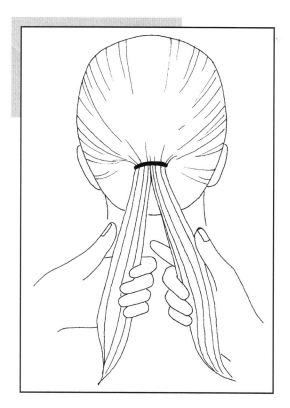

1. Divide ponytail into 2 sections.

2. Take a small section from behind the left-side section.

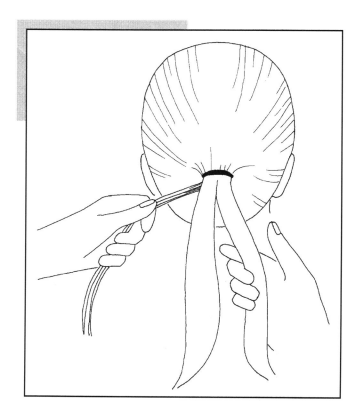

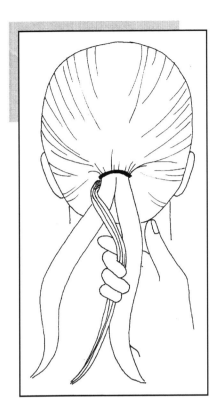

3. Give it to the right side.

4. While holding ponytail securely with the left thumb, and allowing the right side to hang free, take a small section from behind the right side.

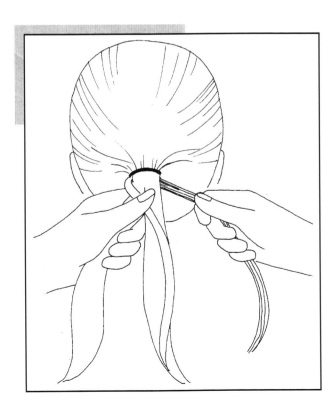

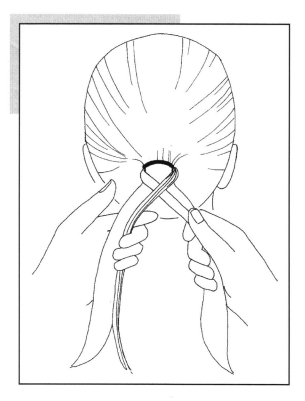

5. Give it to the left side.

6. While holding the right side securely with your right thumb, continue steps 2 through 6 until you reach the end of the ponytail. Secure with a rubberband.

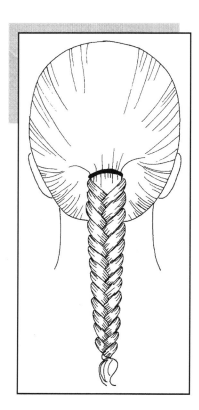

Fishtail

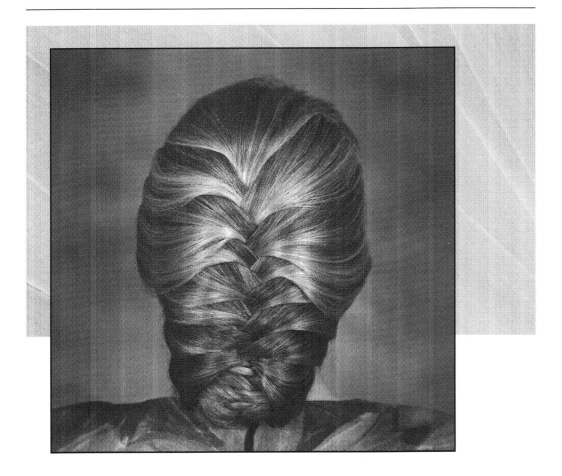

We are going to take the technique you learned in the fishtail ponytail and add to it to create the fishtail braid, which starts in the bang area. If you have perfected the ponytail technique, you will be doing this braid in no time at all. The fishtail is best done on dry, non-layered hair, shoulder length or longer. It is guaranteed to be one of your favorites.

| TIP! | *Make an X. When you pick up one side, make sure you give it to the opposite side.* |

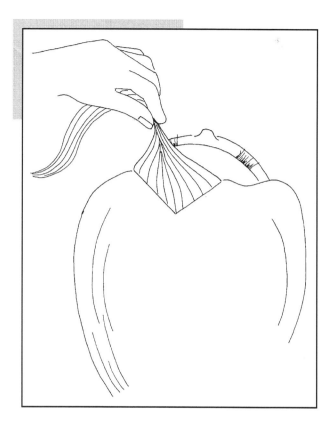

1. Take a triangle section of hair from the front. If there are bangs, begin behind them.

2. Divide this section into 2 strands.

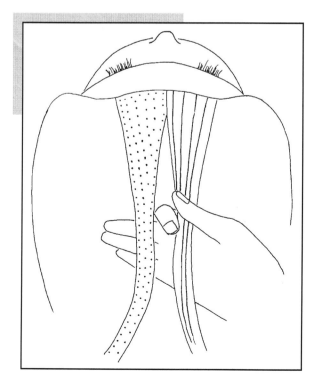

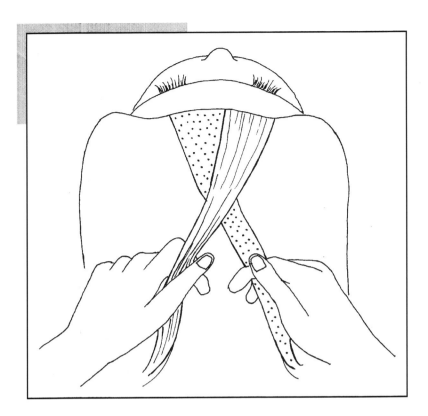

3. Cross the right strand over the left strand.

4. Place both strands in the right hand with the index finger in between, hand palm up, as shown.

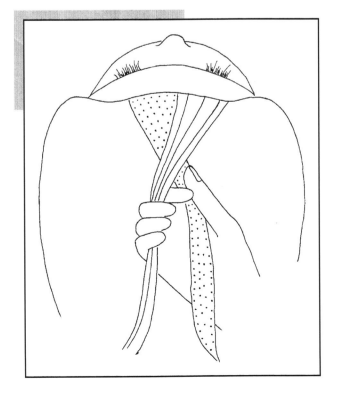

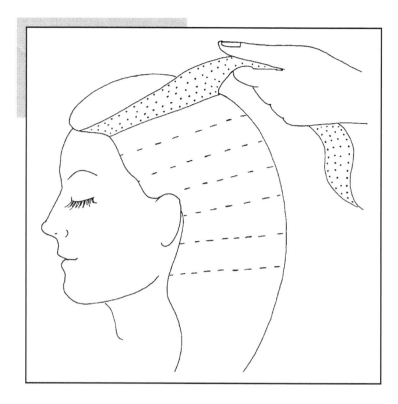

5. Pick up a 1" section on the left side. Starting at the hairline, continue across the head and end in the middle by your right hand.

6. Cross this section over the left strand and add to the right strand. (This makes one side of an *X*.)

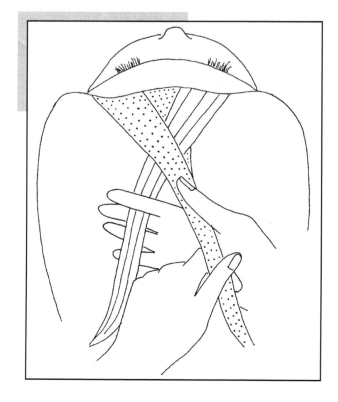

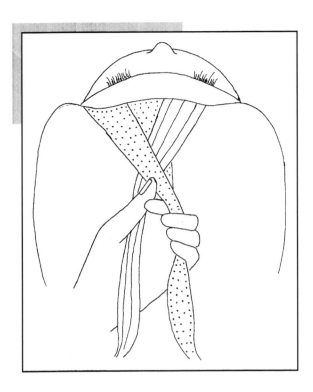

7. Put both strands in the left hand with the index finger in between, hand palm up, as shown.

8. Pick up a 1" section on the right side. Starting at the hairline, continue across the head and end in the middle by your left hand.

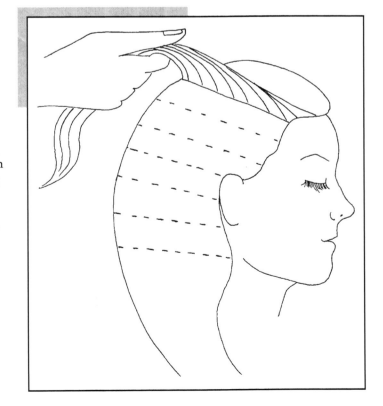

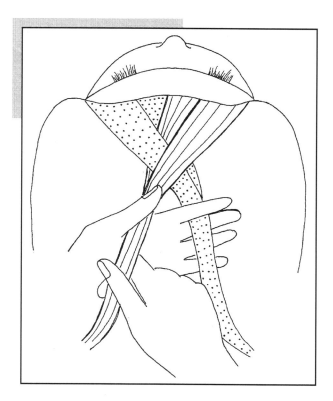

9. Cross the section over the right strand and add it to the left strand. (This makes the other side of the *X*.)

10. Put both strands in the right hand with index finger in between, hand palm up, as shown.

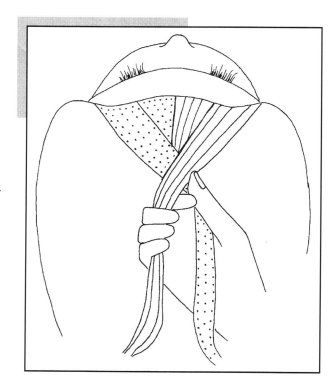

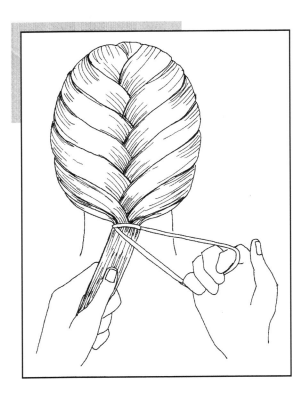

11. Repeat steps 5 through 10, allowing your hand to move down to the nape with each 1" section picked up. When you run out of sections, secure braid with a rubberband.

12. Another option is to keep your hands elevated, at crown level, while you are doing this braid. Once you are finished, but before you put the rubberband in the hair, let your hands relax to the nape area and allow the braid to slide down. This technique creates fullness behind the ears. Finish off the ponytail with the fishtail ponytail technique, and then tuck under and secure with bobby pins. The finished style will look like this.

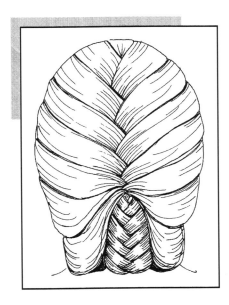

French Braid

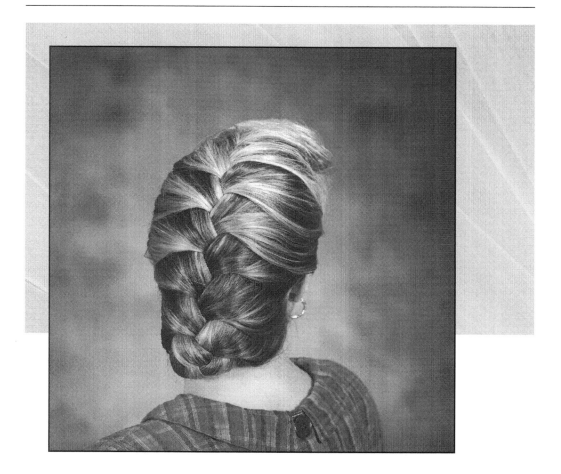

We are now beginning the 3-strand braids. To make them easier to learn, pay special attention to the hand positions, and copy them exactly. This will take the confusion out of working with 3 strands of hair at one time.

Once you have perfected the 3-strand techniques, you are unlimited in the number of different styles you can create. By varying the direction or the number of braids, you can create completely different looks. For example, put a French braid on the left side and then one on the right side. Rubberband them together with a ponytail hanging in the back. Or try doing a Dutch braid, but start it in the nape area instead of the bang area.

The French braid is the braid most requested in salons and is always in style. It can be done on layered or all one-length hair. If it is done on layered hair, it is best to dampen and gel the hair before braiding it. If the style is done on all one-length hair, it is best done with the hair dry.

> **TIP!** *The French braid is done by passing the outside strands over the center strands.*

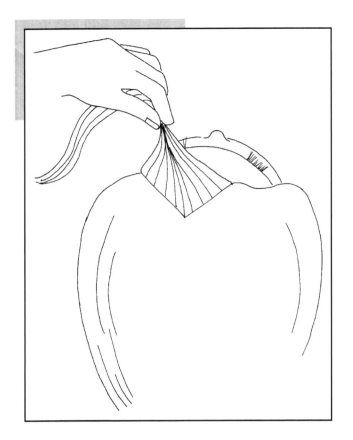

1. Take a triangle section of hair from the front. If there are bangs, begin behind them.

2. Divide this section into 3 strands.

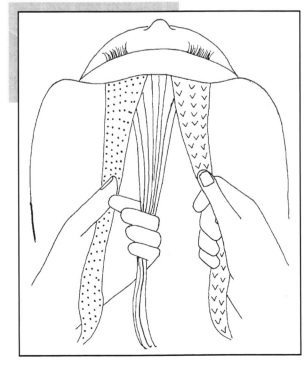

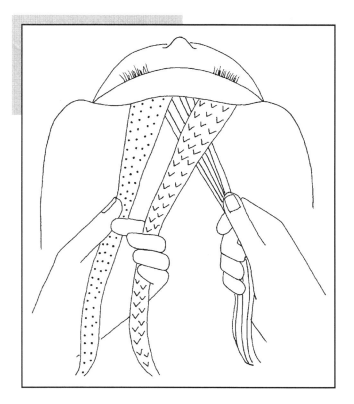

3. Cross the right strand over the center strand.

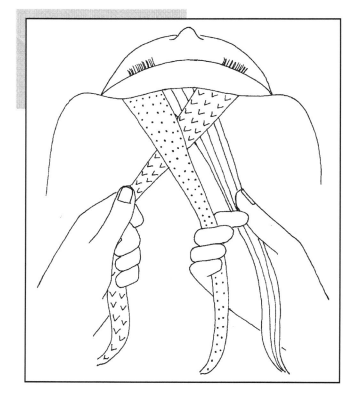

4. Cross the left strand over the center strand.

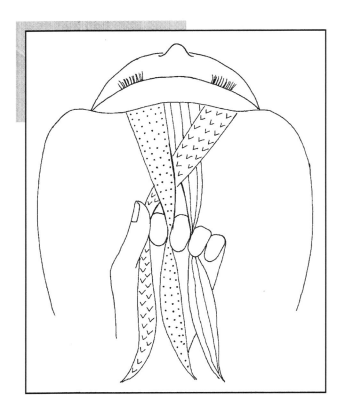

5. Place all 3 strands in left hand, with fingers in between the sections, hand palm up, as shown.

6. Pick up a 1" section on the right side.

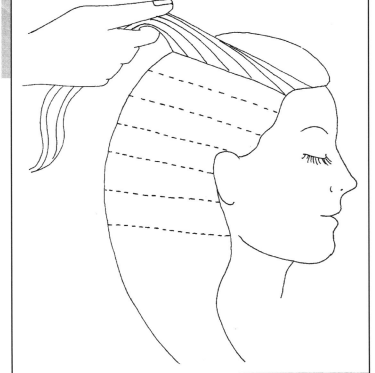

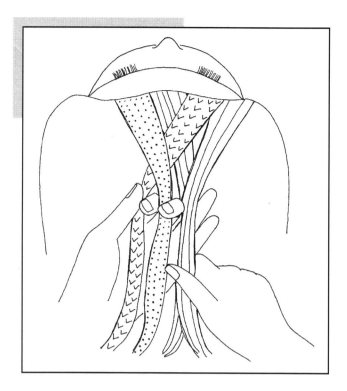

7. Add this section to the right strand already in your hand.

8. Cross right strand over center.

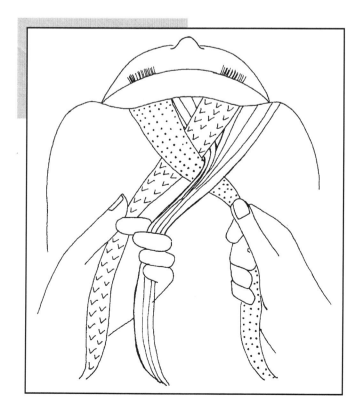

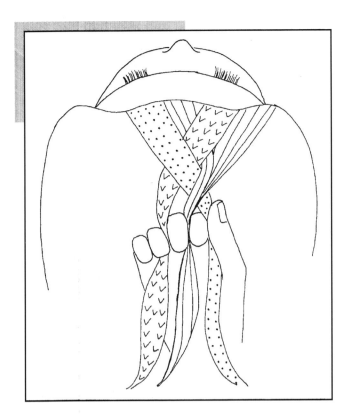

9. Place strands in right hand, fingers in between, hand palm up, as shown.

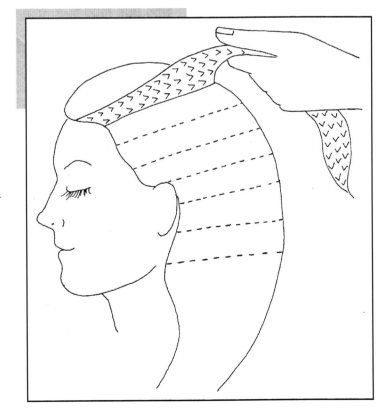

10. Pick up a 1" section on the left side.

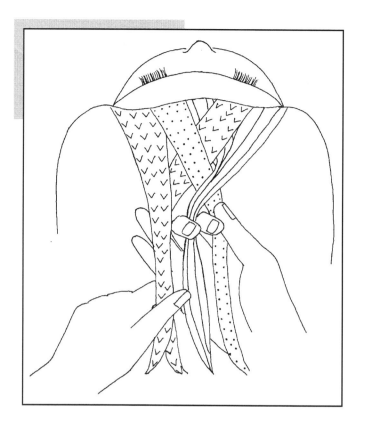

11. Add this section to the left strand already in your hand.

12. Cross the left strand over center strand.

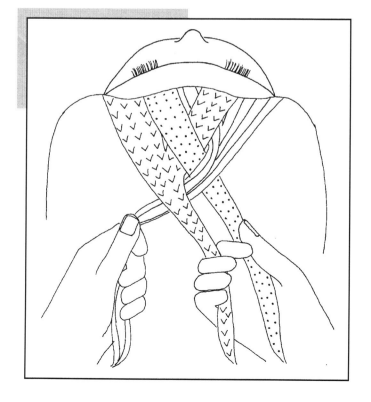

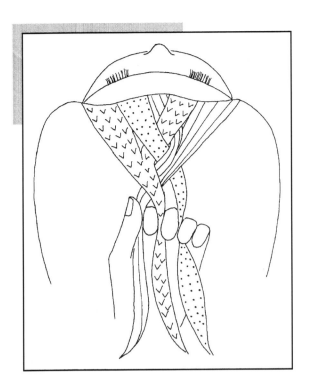

13. Place strands in left hand, fingers in between, hand palm up, as shown.

14. Repeat steps 6 through 13, moving down the nape with each 1" section picked up. When you run out of sections, secure braid with rubberband. Remainder of the hair forms ponytail.

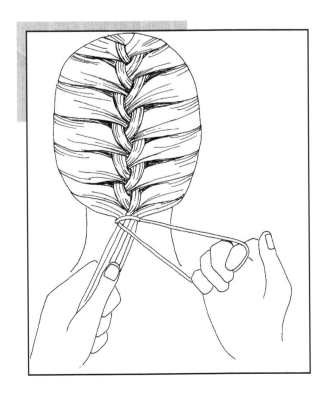

15. Another option is to finish the ponytail by braiding to the ends, as shown.

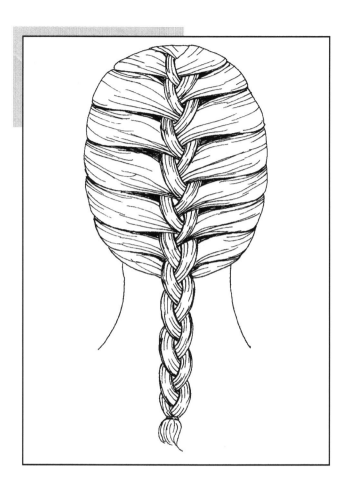

Dutch Braid

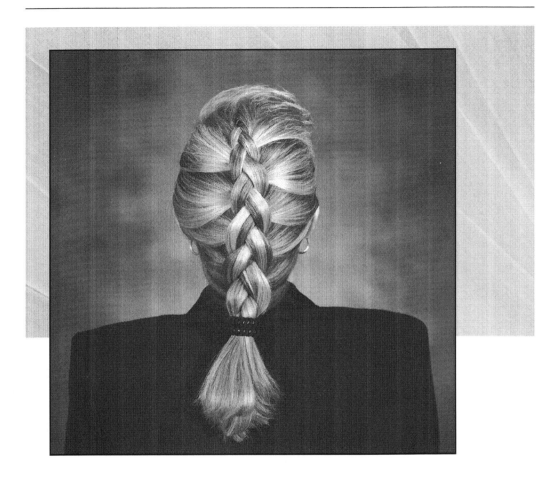

The Dutch braid is very similar to the French braid. The technique is similar, too. It differs only in that, for the Dutch braid, you pass the strands under the center sections instead of over. The Dutch braid can be done on layered or all one-length hair. If it is done on layered hair, it is best to dampen and gel the hair before braiding it. If the style is done on all one-length hair, it is best done with the hair dry.

| **TIP!** | *The Dutch braid is done by crossing the outside strands under the center strands.* |

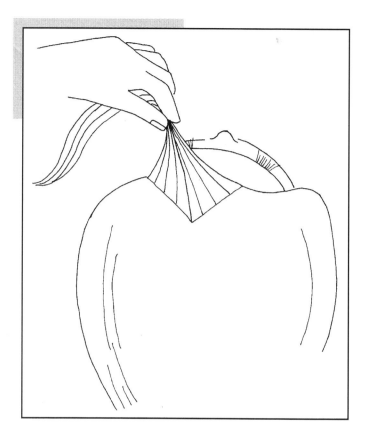

1. Take a triangle section of hair from the front. If there are bangs, begin behind them.

2. Divide this section into 3 strands.

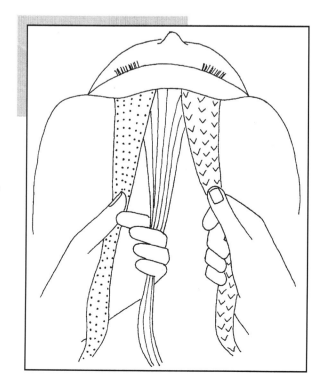

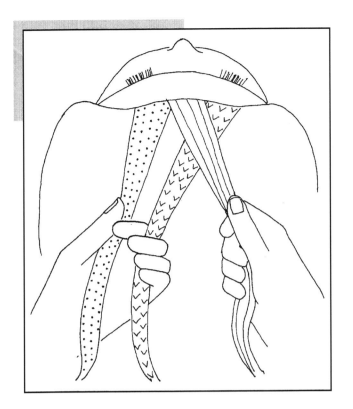

3. Cross the right strand under the center strand.

4. Cross the left strand under the center strand.

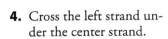
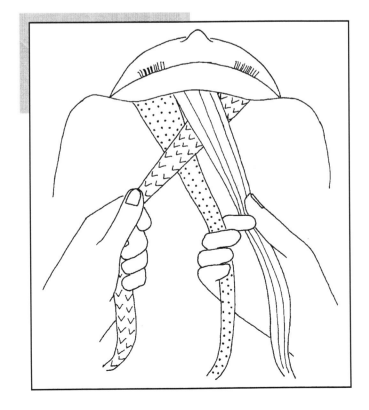

5. Place all 3 strands in left hand, with fingers between the sections, hand palm up, as shown.

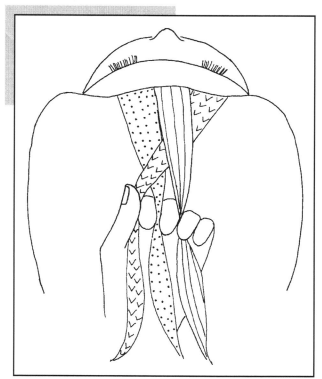

6. Pick up a 1" section on the right side.

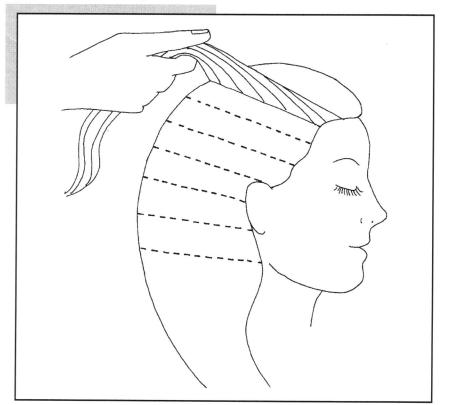

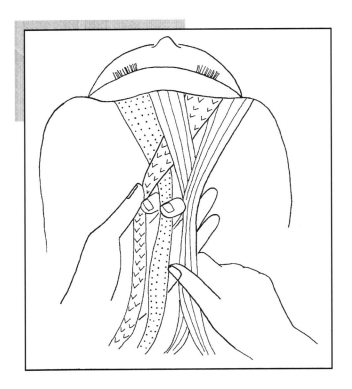

7. Add this section to the right strand already in your hand.

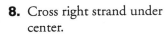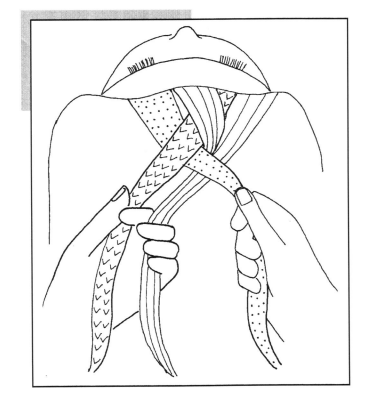

8. Cross right strand under center.

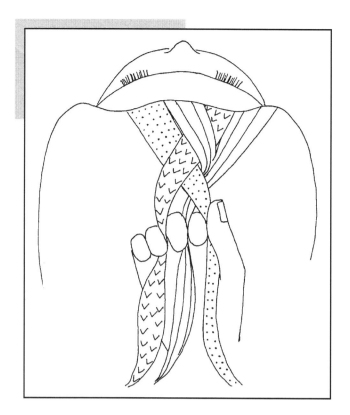

9. Place strands in right hand, fingers in between, hand palm up, as shown.

10. Pick up a 1" section on the left side.

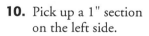

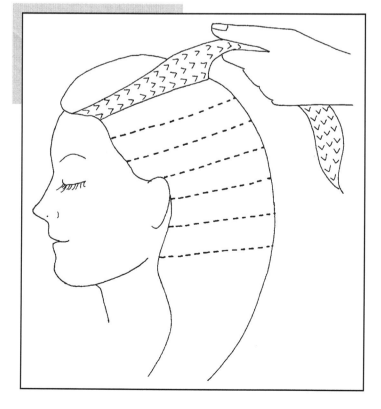

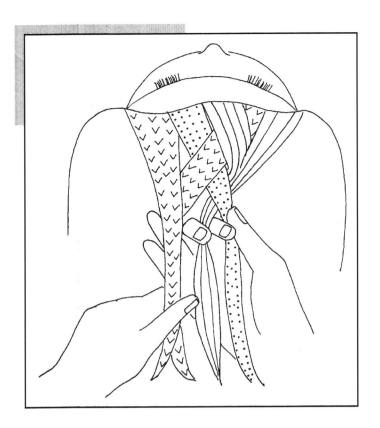

11. Add this section to the left strand already in your hand.

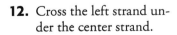

12. Cross the left strand under the center strand.

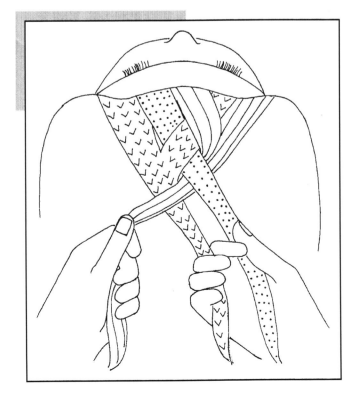

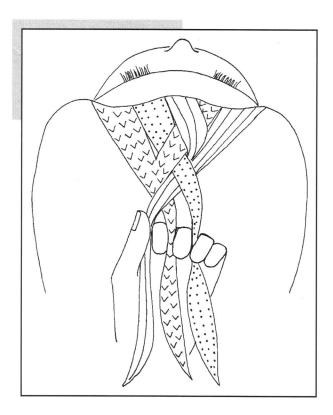

13. Place strands in left hand, fingers in between, hand palm up, as shown.

14. Repeat steps 6 through 13, moving down the nape with each 1" section picked up. When you run out of sections, secure braid with rubberband. Remainder of hair forms ponytail.

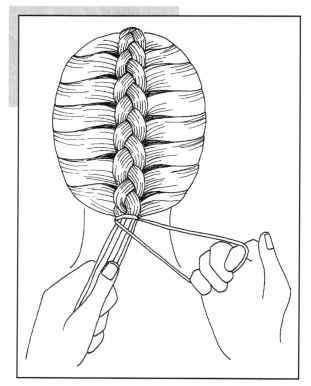

15. Another option is to finish the ponytail by braiding to the ends, as shown.

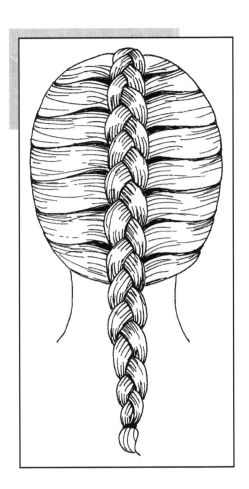

Twisting

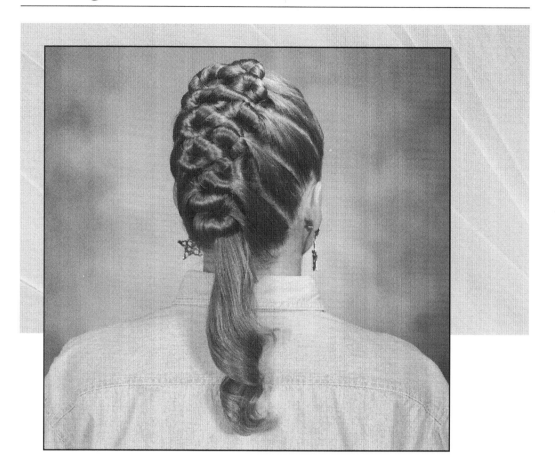

The twisting techniques shown here can be used in varied ways. Following are instructions for forming the twisted design into many figure 8s. But don't think this is the only way to do twisting. It is also very beautiful to allow the twist to be free form and lie where it may.

TIP!   *Be certain the 1" section you are picking up passes over the existing strand, not under it.*

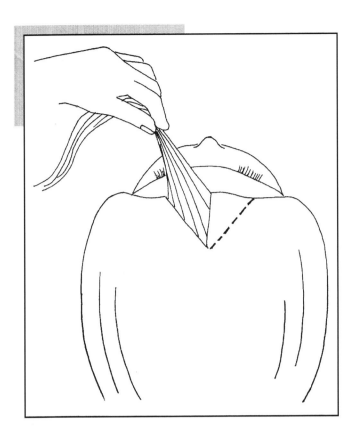

1. Take a triangle section just to the left side of center. If there are bangs, begin behind them.

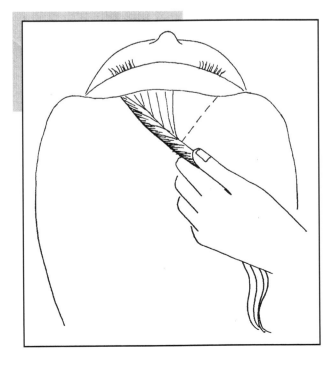

2. Begin twisting this section of hair toward the right and move your body over by the person's right shoulder.

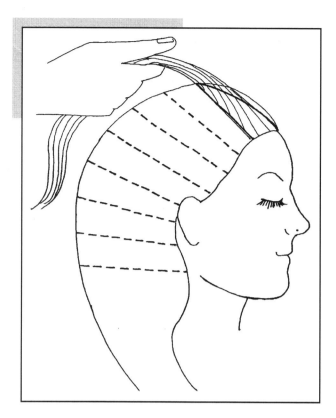

3. Pick up a 1" section on the right side.

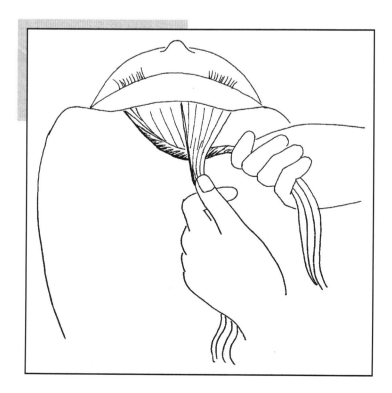

4. Take this new strand and pass it over the top of the twisted strand.

5. Continue wrapping this new strand in a counterclockwise direction around the twisted strand until they become one strand.

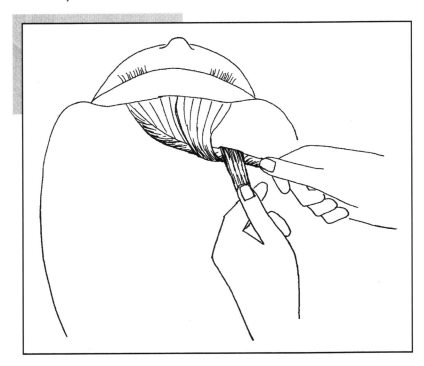

6. As you walk to the left shoulder, force the twisted strand up to form the top part of an 8.

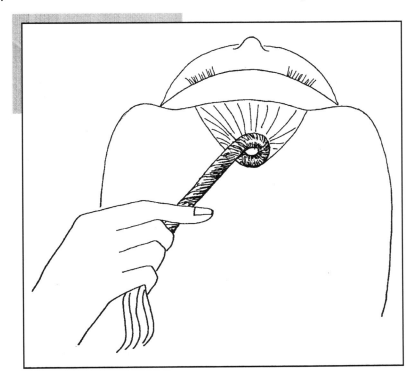

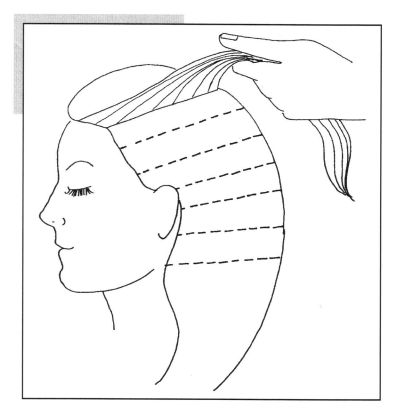

7. Pick up a 1" section on the left side.

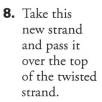

8. Take this new strand and pass it over the top of the twisted strand.

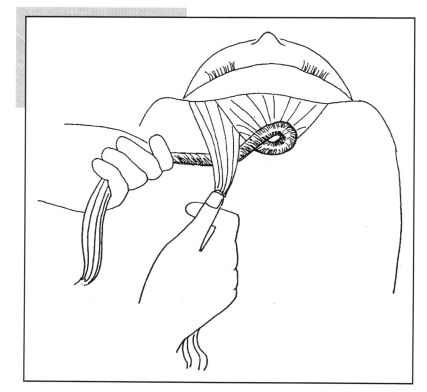

9. Continue wrapping this new strand in a clockwise direction around the twisted strand until they make one strand.

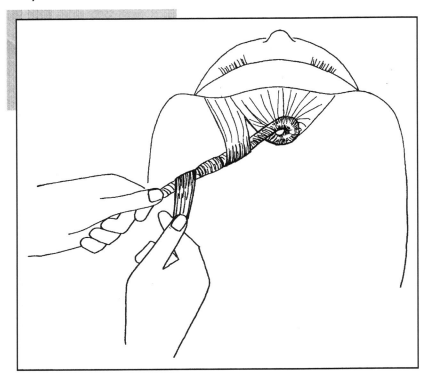

10. As you walk to the right shoulder, force the twisted strand up to form the bottom part of an 8.

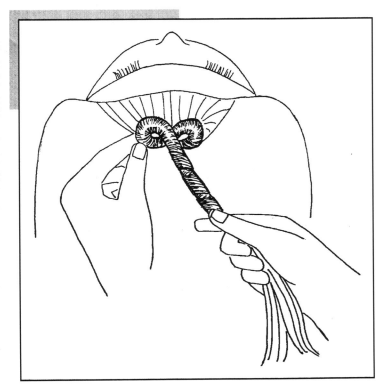

11. Repeat steps 3 through 10, moving down toward the nape with each 1" section picked up. When you run out of sections, secure the twist with bobby pins. You might want to softly curl the piece of remaining hair and place it over the person's shoulder.

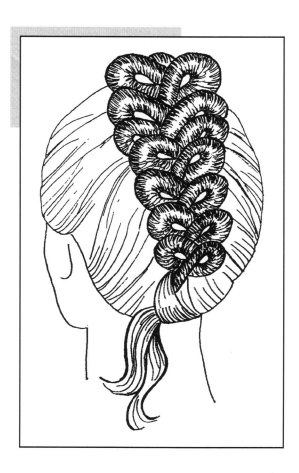

Knotting

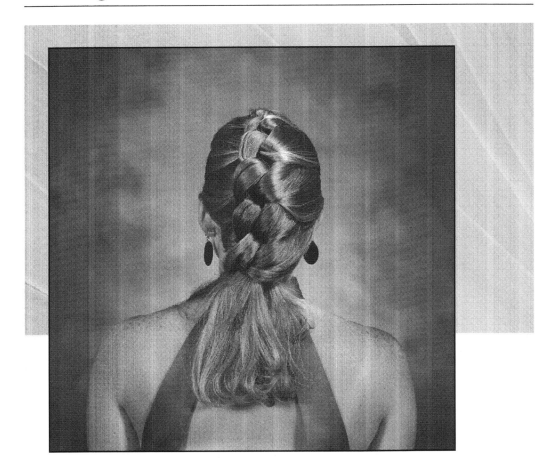

This style is easy and fun to do. People always ask how it's done because it looks so complicated. But as you have already learned, just because you can't figure out how it's done by looking at it doesn't mean it is difficult to do. The key to knotting is that it's best done on dry, all one-length hair.

TIP! *You must tie the knots exactly the same each time. If you tie right over left, as we have done here, you must follow through and tie it that way each time.*

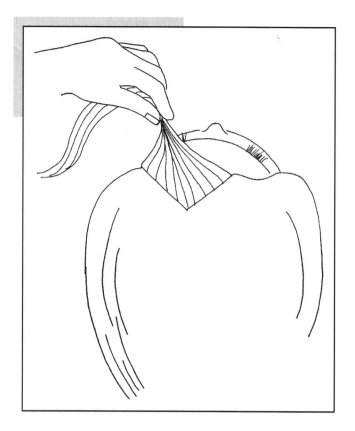

1. Make a triangle section at the top. If there are bangs, begin behind them.

2. Divide this section into 2 strands.

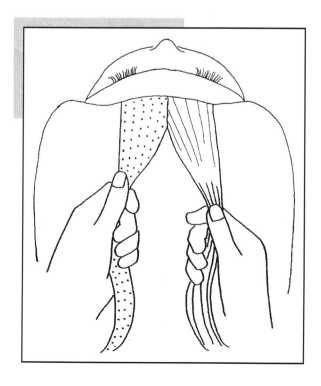

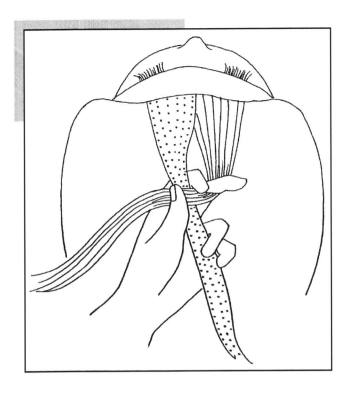

3. Place both sections in your left hand, matching the hand positions shown. Then, place the right strand over the left strand.

4. Using your right thumb and index finger, reach between the strands and pull the right strand through the 2 strands.

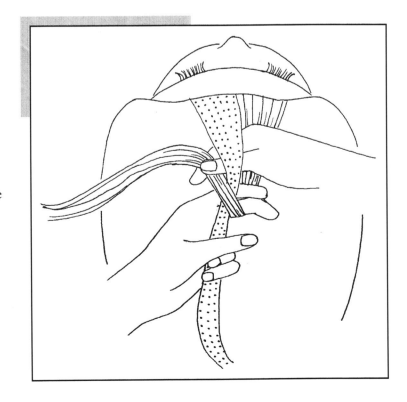

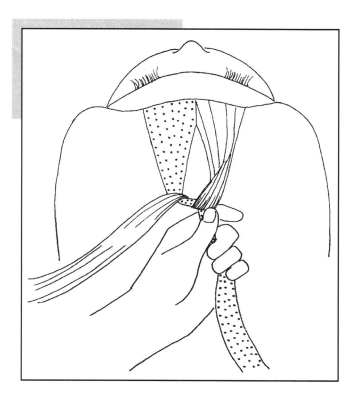

5. Make sure the strand you pulled between the 2 strands is kept to the left side.

6. Pull both strands so the hair ties next to the scalp. You have just tied the first part of a knot.

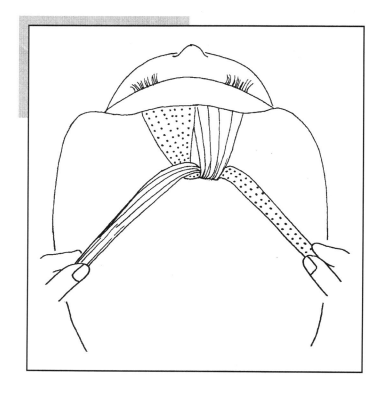

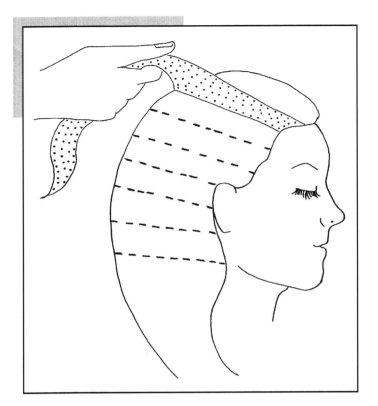

7. Place both strands in the left hand, fingers in between. Pick up a 1" section on the right side of the head.

8. Add this section to the right-side section already in your hand.

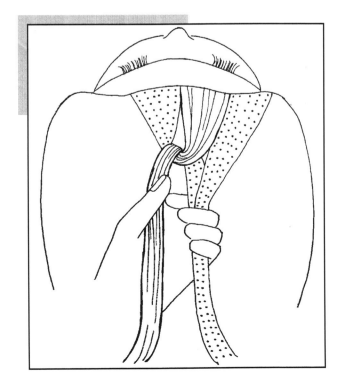

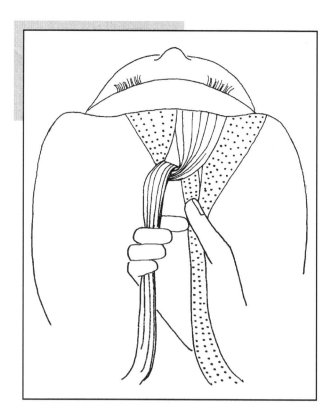

9. Place both sections in your right hand, finger in between as shown. (You have just changed hands.)

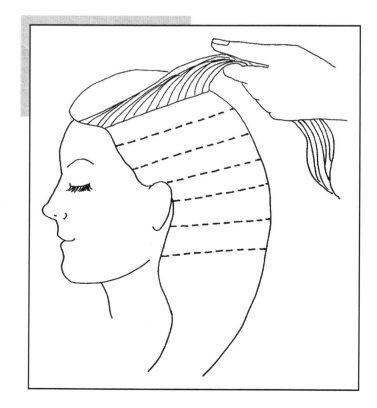

10. Pick up a 1" section on the left side of the head.

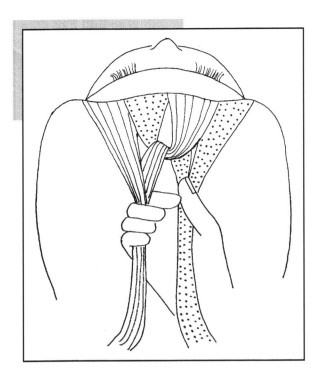

11. Add it to the left-side section already in your hand.

12. Repeat steps 3 through 11, picking up 1" sections as you move down the head. Continue until you reach the nape and run out of sections to pick up. Tie the 2 strands together a few more times, and then roll under and pin. Curl remaining tendrils with a curling iron and rest over shoulder.

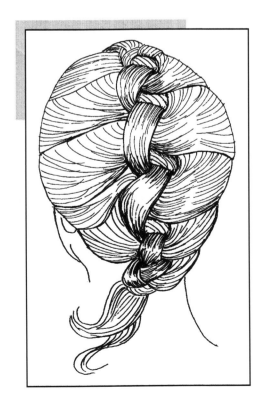

The Bow

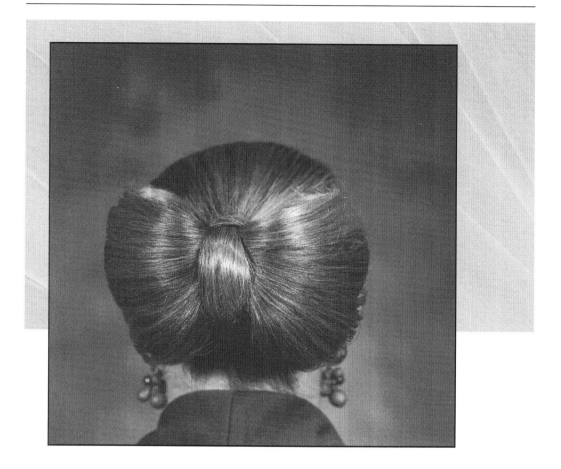

Everyone should know how to make a bow. It is such an elegant evening look. Following are instructions for making a bow very easily. See if you don't agree.

> **TIP!** *Be sure to cover the rubberband with hair or a hair accessory before you make the bow. It is too difficult to cover later.*

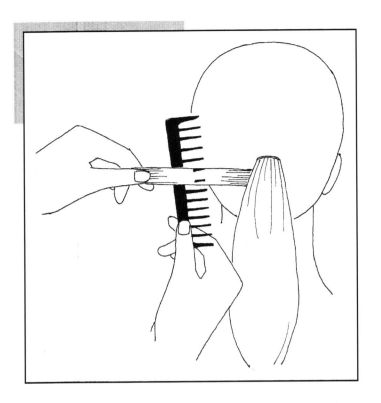

1. Make a ponytail where you want the center of the bow to be positioned. Take a small section from underneath the pony-tail and back-comb.

2. Wrap this back-combed section around rub-berband and secure with hairpins.

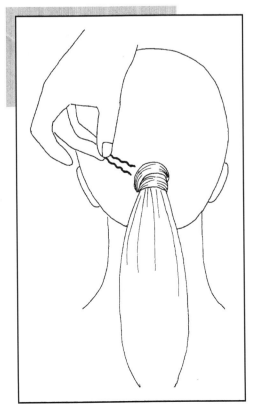

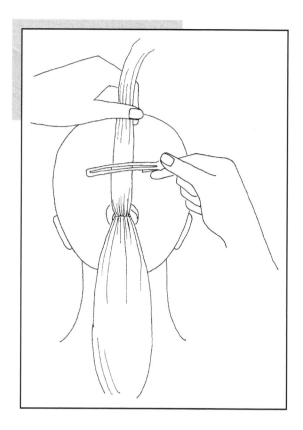

3. Remove a small section from the
top of ponytail and clip up out of
your way.

4. Divide remaining ponytail
into 2 sections.

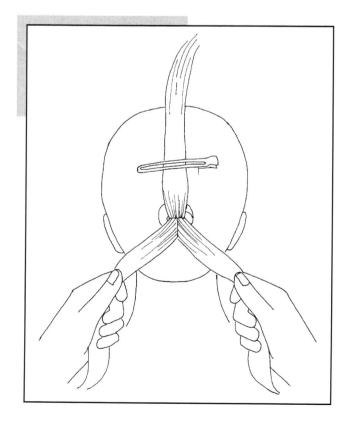

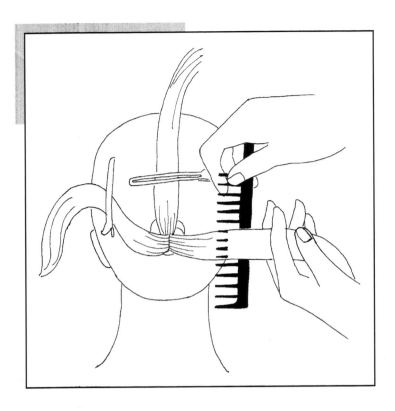

5. Clip left side out of your way. Back-comb the right side, making sure to hold hair straight out to the side as shown.

6. Roll back-combed section into a barrel curl, placing it behind the right ear. Secure with bobby pins. Use your fingers to fan out barrel curl to make it as wide as possible without splitting. Use hairpins to tack in place. This is the finished right side of your bow.

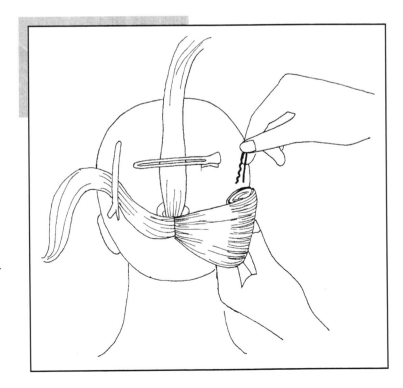

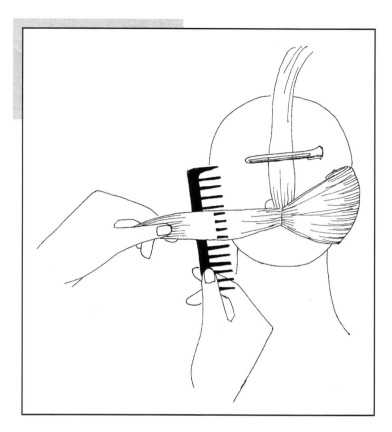

7. Next, back-comb left side and roll into a barrel curl, placing it behind the left ear. Secure with bobby pins and fan out the barrel curl with your fingers, making it as wide as possible.

8. Take the small section you clipped out of your way in step 3 and gently back-comb. Roll this section into a pin curl. Lay this section over the split in the ponytail and bobby pin the curl underneath.

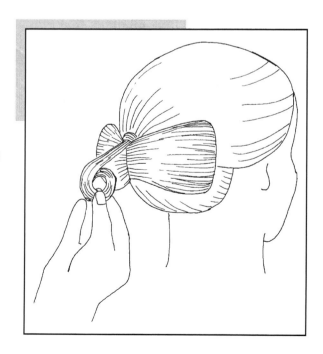

9. The finished bow will look like this. Make sure to use a finishing spray to keep smooth and fixed in place.

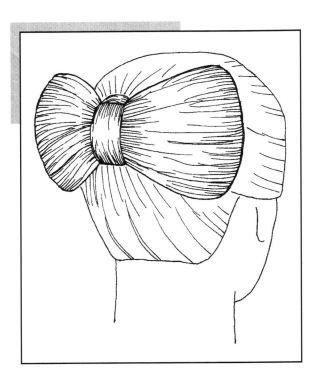

The Bowtie

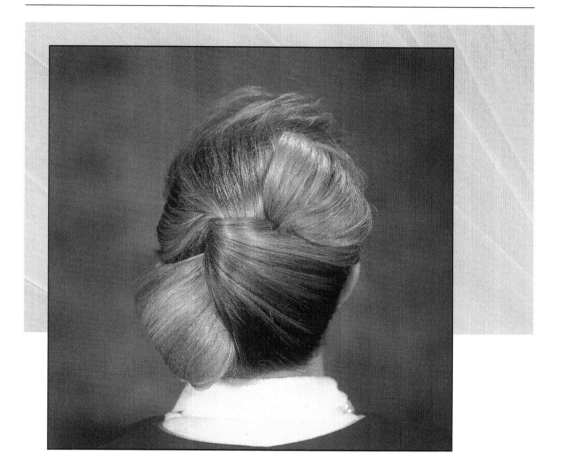

The bowtie is a beautiful finished style as well as a perfect base for many different long hair designs. It is recommended that you become comfortable tying this style, and then experiment with the ponytail pieces to create a completely different style. Have fun with the different options this style gives you.

The bowtie is best done on dry, all one-length hair. When first learning how to tie this style, you may find it easier to make it neat if you dampen and gel the hair first. This stops the strands from wrinkling when tied. If you are working with dampened hair, back-combing is not recommended.

| TIP! | *The right-hand side must tie over, then under, the left side and end up at the crown.* |

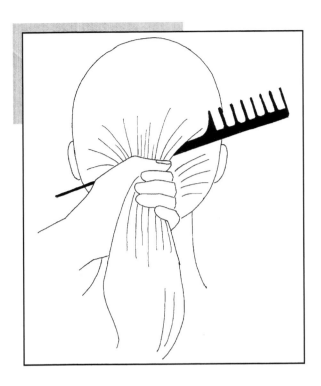

1. Comb the hair back into a ponytail and hold it with your left hand. Using a tail comb, make a diagonal section along the scalp, starting at the top of the right ear and ending behind the bottom of the left ear.

2. Put your comb down and place the right section in your right hand and the left section in your left hand.

   Hint: Try to copy the hand positions exactly on steps 3 and 4. This will take the confusion out of trying to manipulate these sections without the hair's getting messy.

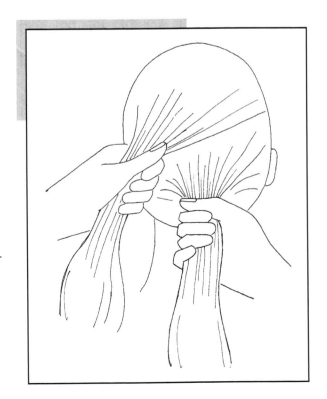

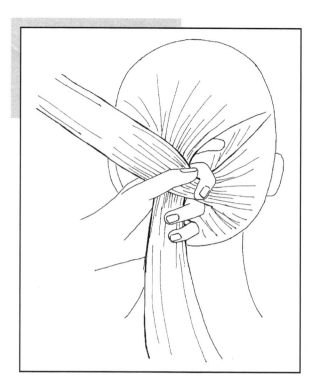

3. Using your thumb, index finger, and third finger to keep these sections separated, place the right section over the left section.

4. Reach through the strand separation and grab the strand on top. Pull it through and toward the crown.

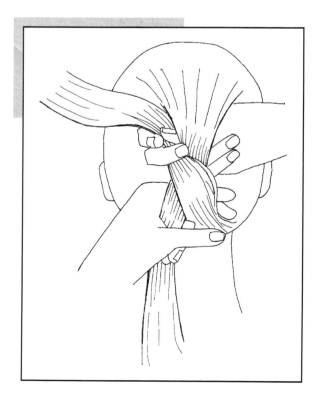

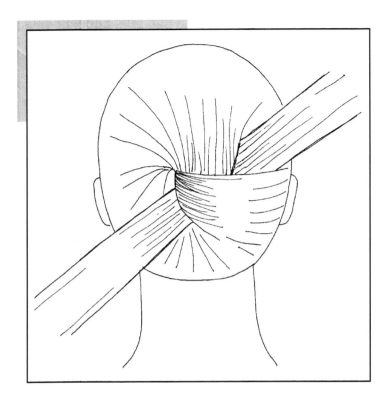

5. You have just tied the hair.

6. Using bobby pins, make sure you securely fasten the tied section of the hair. This is very important. If it is not securely pinned, the entire style can slide out.

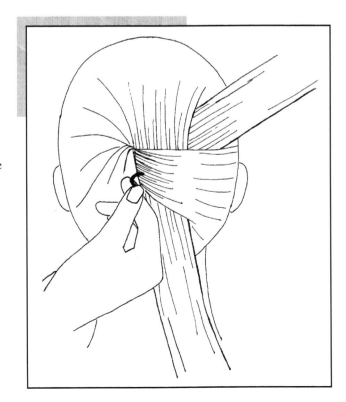

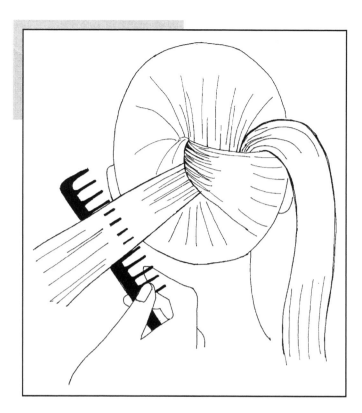

7. Taking the section on the left, lightly back-comb it while directing the section to behind the left ear.

8. Roll this section under into a barrel curl and bobby pin into place. After pinning it, spread this curl out as wide as you feel is necessary.

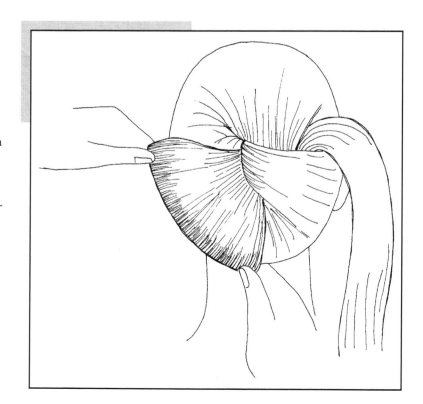

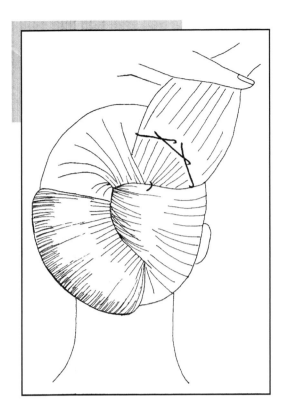

9. Lightly back-comb the top section, direct it forward toward the face, and bobby pin as shown.

10. Make a barrel curl, rolling back away from the face. Bobby pin this curl as close to the tied section as possible. Spread this curl as needed and use bobby pins to tack in place.

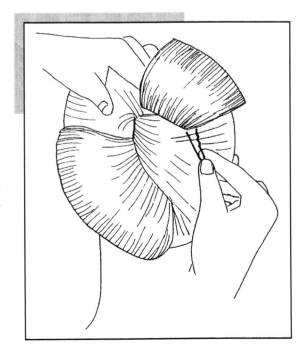

11. This is the finished style.

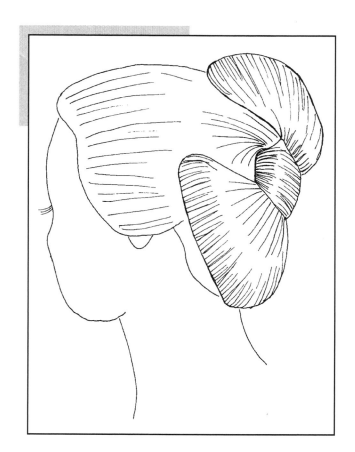

French Twist

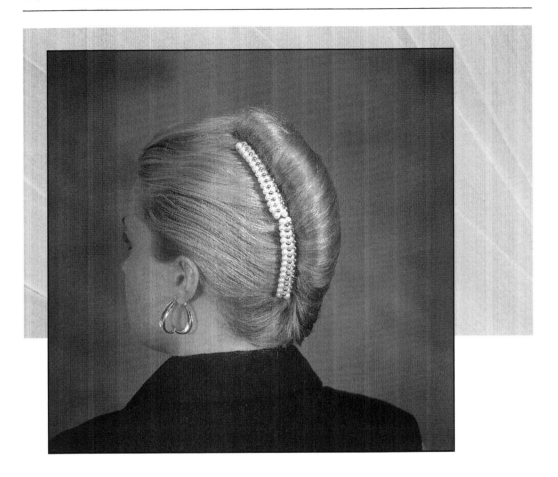

Following are instructions for the easiest way found to do the French twist. There is no back-combing and no setting. The French twist is a simple, smooth look with no fullness around the face. The technique will require practice, but once you have perfected it, you will use it often.

| TIP! | *The hand positions are easily copied when you stand in front of the person's right shoulder.* |

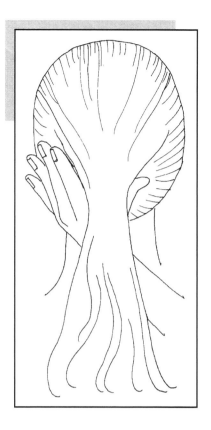

1. Comb the hair back into a ponytail and hold it with your left hand, palm facing toward nape with hand in a *V* position as shown.

2. Close fingers together, making sure to keep hand in the closed *V* position. Do not close hand into a circle as with a ponytail.

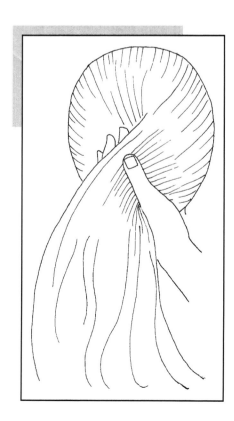

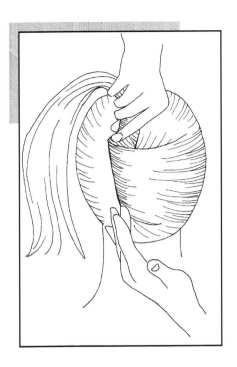

3. Reaching over the person's head with your right arm, grab the hair strand and begin wisting the entire strand to your right.

4. Continue loosely twisting the strand until you have reached the ends of the hair.

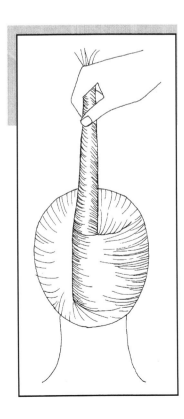

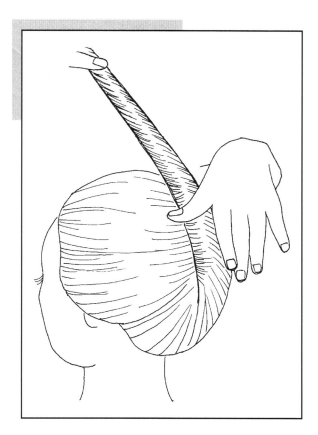

5. Place your left thumb against the head in the crown area.

6. Bring the twisted strand down toward the nape, and back up again if necessary, so all the hair is folded together.

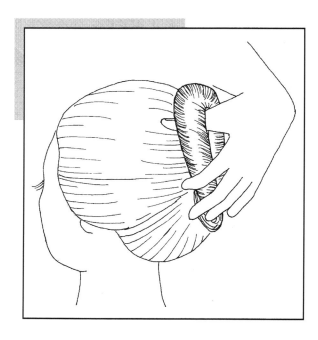

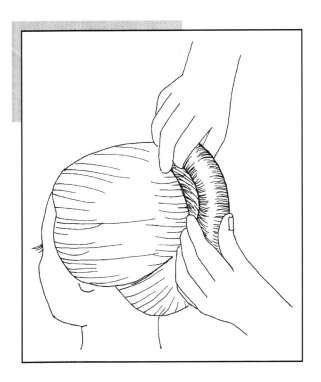

7. Take this folded hair and tuck it under the beginning twist.

8. Secure along twist with bobby pins and hairpins.

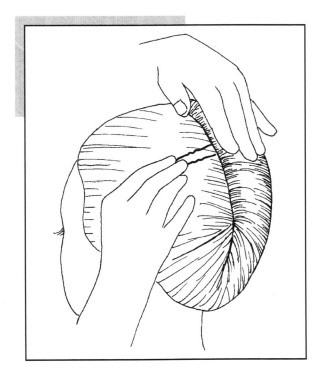

9. This is the finished style.

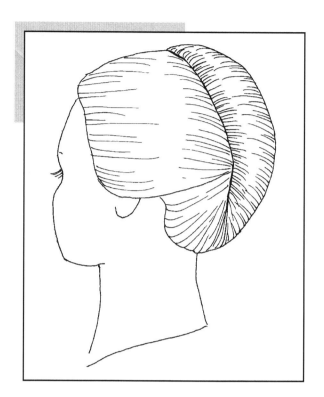

CHAPTER 3

Curls, Kinks, and Coils: Working with Texture

INTRODUCTION

There is no such thing as "good" hair or "bad" hair. This chapter focuses on traditional braiding, locking, and twisting hairstyles that create an aesthetic look for all hair textures. Many of these styles are cultural in origin, as they are derived from traditional African braiding designs that date back to ancient dynasties. The following descriptions will provide you with the basic knowledge of the popular natural braid styles and techniques. The creative art form is unlimited, and the techniques offered here are fundamental and can be improvised to allow self-expression.

CORNROWS

There are many techniques for starting the traditional on-the-base braid known as the cornrow. The cornrow is created with a 3-strand, on-the-scalp braid, which uses an underhand "pick-up" technique. The fundamentals of braiding start with the basic cornrow. According to master braid designer Annu Prestonia, co-owner of Khamit Kinks in New York and Georgia and celebrity braid designer (among her clients are such notables as Stevie Wonder and Angela Basset), cornrows are the foundation of all braid styles. "If you excel at the art of cornrowing, all other braiding techniques are at your disposal," says Prestonia.

To cornrow like a professional you must be patient and practice. A skilled braider must take the time daily to practice cornrowing. Cornrowing is the repetition of the entire woven patterns; the sequence of weave patterns may vary and will determine the style. However, the series of revolutions is a simple repetition of a secure pick-up motion. Practicing will help you to develop speed, accuracy, and finger/wrist dexterity. The time required for braiding can vary from 2 hours for a large braid to 2 days for a micro braid. Mastering the basic cornrow technique will enable you to approach other braid styles with confidence.

Skillful cornrowing is designed through the process of sculpting the parted sections. Sculpting is more than just vertical or horizontal partings. When sculpting the braid, you must first visualize the finished look. This will allow you to create smooth and consistent curved partings that contour with the head. The curved partings are a part of the design, so they must be neat and even. The more creative you are in designing the parts, the more beautiful the finished sculpted look will be. This contouring, or sculpting, is especially beautiful on small to medium sized cornrows.

Three-Strand Cornrow

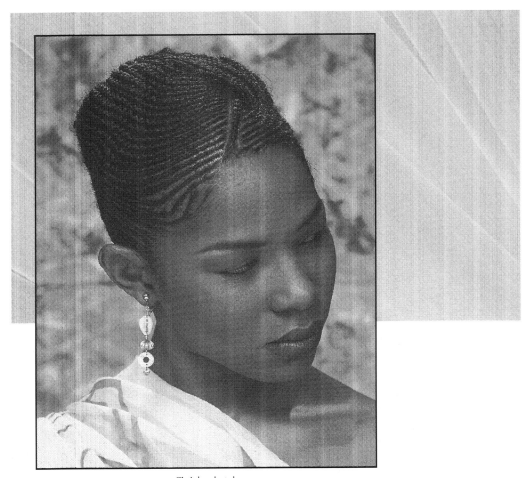

Finished style

Practice the following technique for cornrowing. It uses 3 strands with an underhand weaving motion, in which the strands on the sides are always passed under the center strand, alternating between the right side and the left. Tulani Kinard, master braider and owner of Tulani's Regal Movement in New York, gives the following technique:

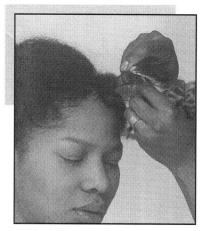

Divide the hair into equal parts.

1. Begin by taking a section as small as you want the braid to be. Divide the section into 3 equal strands. Start at the hairline (depending on the style, the braid can begin anywhere from the nape of the neck forward). The strand on the far left will be called strand 1, the center is strand 2, and the strand on the far right is strand 3.

2. Cross left strand 1 under center strand 2. Center strand 2 is now on the left, and strand 1 is the new center. Passing the strand under the center with each revolution creates the underhand cornrow braid.

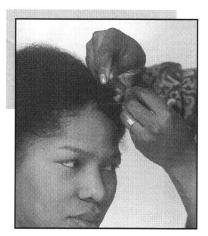

Cross strand 1 underneath strand 2.

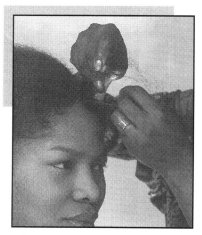

3. With each crossing under, or revolution, you must pick up new equal size sections of hair and add them to center strand 2; pick up before crossing the outer strands under the center strand. Now cross strand 3 under strand 1. At the end of this revolution, strand 3 is the new center.

Cross strand 3 under strand 1.

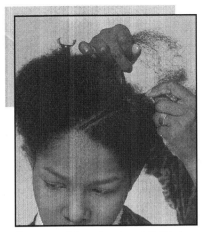

Pass strand 2 under strand 3. Work from side to side.

4. Each time you make a revolution (crossing under the center strand), you must pick up the hair from the scalp and add it to the new center. With each revolution, alternate the side of the braid on which you pick up hair.

5. As you move along the section, cornrowing and picking up more hair, you add fullness to the braid. Contoured parting should be clean and neat.

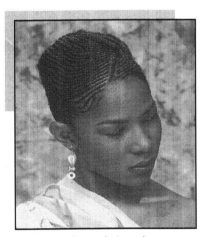

Finished style: Sculpting—the three-strand cornrow.

Cornrows with Extension

Hair additions, or extensions, are used for the following reasons:

- To lengthen short hair.
- To add volume to thin hair.
- To protect damaged hair.
- To add dimension to the height of the natural hair.
- To allow the braid style to last longer.
- To make a creative and cultural statement.

Cornrow with Extension (Feed-in Method)

The feed-in method can be applied to cornrows or individual braids. There are several different methods for integrating extension hair into the hairline. Some methods just introduce large amounts of extension material into the fragile hairline, leaving the front of the braid bulky and knotted. In some cases, this bulky, bumpy look has become very popular. These are fast and effective methods for adding extensions if you don't mind the braids looking like a helmet!

But many braid professionals contend that the braid extension should be concealed and the knot or lump eliminated because it is damaging to the hair. "When hair is braided using the knot or lump at the beginning of the braid, it is a tell-tale sign that you are wearing an extension," notes Taliah Waajid, author of *Hairitage Masterpieces.* She uses the feed-in method to gradually add hair throughout the braid. Literally, strand by strand the braid must be built up. Too large amounts of extension material place excessive weight on the fragile areas of the hairline. They also tighten and pull the hair and create an unrealistic finished look. By properly applying the correct amount of tension with the feed-in method, you can eliminate the artificial look.

The traditional cornrow does not look like a hat of braids. It is flat, natural, and contoured to the scalp. The parting is definitely important because it defines the finished style. The feed-in method creates a tapered, or narrow, base at the hairline. As small pieces, or strips, of extension hair are added, the base fills in, which brings the adjoining braids closer together.

This technique takes longer to perform. However, the cornrow lasts longer, looks more natural, and does not put excessive tension on the hairline. Practice this method for a flat contour, natural cornrow style.

The Feed-in Method

1. Start at the hairline by parting off a cornrow base in the desired style.

2. At the starting point, no extension is usually added. If the hair extension is required because of the thinning hairline, minute amounts can be applied to 5 to 10 strands. This is all relative to the size of the cornrow.

3. Divide the natural hair into 3 equal portions.

4. With the first revolution, left strand 1 crosses *under* strand 2.

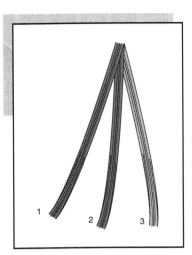

Three-strand extension

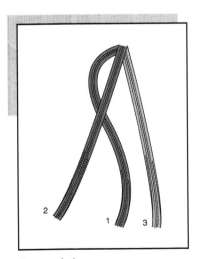

First revolution

5. On the second revolution, right strand 3 crosses *under* strand 1. A small portion of natural hair is picked up and added to the outside portion during the revolution.

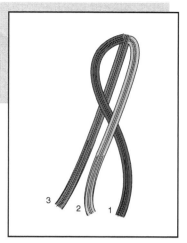

Second revolution

6. On the third revolution, bring strand 3 to the center, picking up a small portion at the base of natural hair.

7. After several revolutions and pick ups, apply small amounts of folded extensions under the natural hair, to the center and outside portions. Hair extension must be tucked into the fold of the 2 adjoining portions. The amount of extension should be proportionately less than the size of the base.

8. The folded extension is always applied to the center and outside portions before the pick up. Do not forget to pick up natural hair with *each* revolution to execute on-the-base cornrow.

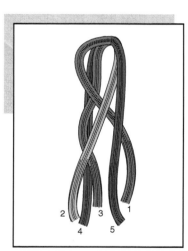

Third revolution

NOTE! *There are several different ways to start a cornrow and feed in extension pieces. Experiment with as many methods as you can. Different hairlines and styles require different methods.*

Over-directing Braid Extension

Precision parting and sectioning is vital to all braiding techniques. Parting will determine the direction of the braid. Clean and precise partings are required to create a strong braid base. Hair strands must never be over-directed or misplaced within an adjacent braid. If single strands are incorporated into another section outside of their own section, the hair will eventually break. Over-extending the hair adds tension to the unsupported strand.

During the cornrow process, when you are picking up hair at the base, the hair directly underneath the previous revolution must be incorporated into the braid. The hair picked up must never come from another subsection or be extended up into the braid from a lower part of the braid.

The same is true when applying any braid technique. When creating an individual braid with extensions, start in the center of the subsection. Over-extending or misplacing the beginning of the extension leaves the hair exposed and unsupported, which can lead to breakage and traction alopecia. This is particularly true when adding extensions to the hairline. If the extension is not secure (2 or 3 revolutions before picking up), the extension will move away from the point of entry. This pulled base around the hairline will definitely create breakage and eventually alopecia.

TIP! *For professional finishing, always trim split ends that may pop through the braid shaft. Hold scissors flat, moving up the braid shaft. Avoid cutting into the braid.*

Senegalese Twists

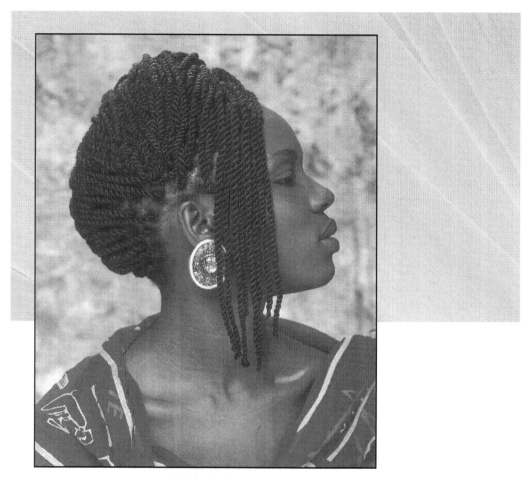

Finished style

Senegalese twists have their origin in West Africa. These braids are created using lin, synthetic material, Kanekalon, or yarn extension material. They use a 2-strand braiding technique. Pre-plan the final style to determine how much material you will need. This will be determined by the length of the desired extension and the size of the partings. Separate and cut to the desired length.

The steps for preparing the hair and scalp are as follows:

1. Shampoo; apply hot oil treatment; blow dry.
2. Match extension material to the person's hair color and texture.

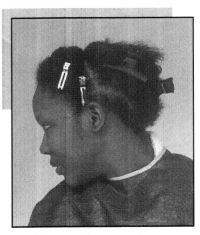

Part hair at 45-degree angle.

1. Start by dividing the entire head of hair in half from ear to ear.

2. Slightly above the ear with tail of comb, make a 45-degree part down toward the neck. The part can be as large or small as required for the size of the twist you are trying to create.

3. Make a subsection above the ear. Separate the subsection into 2 equal parts. Section off a required amount of extension material. Place the extension strip between the 2 equal parts.

4. Simultaneously, you must perform 2 twisting motions. The first twisting is to roll the fiber between both of your fingers, which secures the natural hair into the fiber. The second twisting motion takes the "rolled" fiber and hair and twists, or overlaps, one strand over the other. This rolling motion is done with the fingertip and the roll should be very tight.

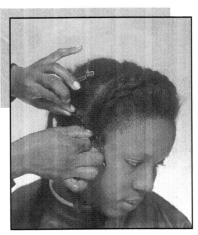

Roll fiber 3 or 4 times.

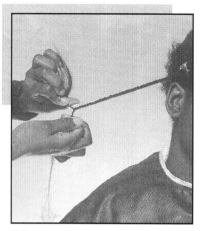

Twist one strand over the other to create a tight twist.

5. Continue the double twist motion for the entire length of the strand. Roll and cross strands until you reach the ends. Loop and knot the twists to close. Trim excess fiber.

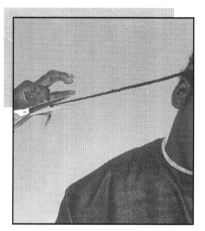

Seal the ends in the predetermined fashion.

6. Seal ends with singeing method or knot and cut close.

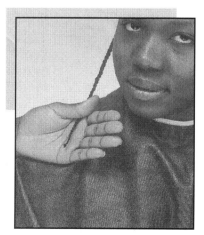

Finished sealed ends

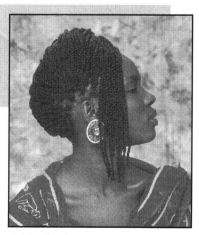

Finished style

Diamond Casama Braids

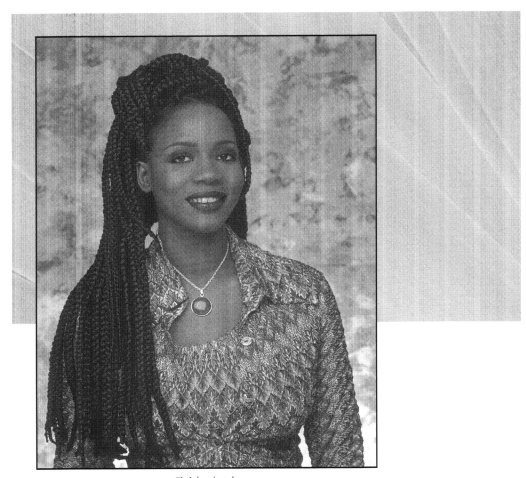

Finished style

Casamas are created by using individual partings and braids that are larger in size than box braids or single braids. This technique requires 3-strand braiding. The stitch of the braid itself is very tight, which allows the braid to curve when finished. The technique begins at the nape, where square, triangular, or rectangular partings are taken in any size desired. For the typical triangular style, triangles are 1/2 to 1". The first 2 or 3 rows from the nape up can be horizontal; when you reach the top, pre-plan your design based on whether or not an asymmetrical look is desired. If it is, create a side part and plan to create braids that begin at the part line and move across the top of the head. This means the partings will follow an angled line and will not be perfectly horizontal at the top.

When the entire head is completed in the desired fashion, the free-hanging braids are singed with a burner. Senior braid stylist Fanta Kaba of Tendrils, New York, performs this technique.

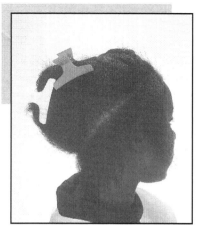

Parting hair at 45-degree angle

1. Start in the back of the head by parting a diagonal section at about a 45-degree angle, toward the front hairline, just past the ear. This section can be from 1 to 2" wide.

2. Part the base into subsections with vertical parts to create the diamond sections. After subsection size has been determined, select the appropriate amount of Kanekalon. For tapered ends, the extension material is gently pulled at both sides so that the ends have a "shredded" uneven effect.

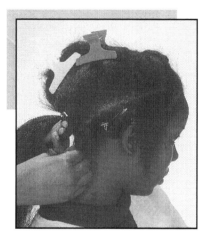

Diagonal sub-partings

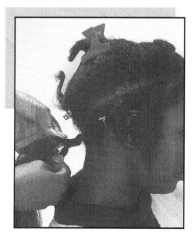

Three-strand braiding

3. Take a strand of synthetic hair of a pre-determined length and fold it in half. Position the center of the strand at the base of the parting and wrap half of the strand 2 or 3 revolutions around the base of the parted natural hair (base wrap is optional).

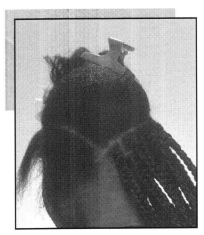

V shape partings

4. Immediately divide the hair into 3 sections, with the natural hair encompassed in the center section. Make certain that the natural hair is concealed under the section before you begin 3-strand braiding.

5. Alternate diagonal partings so that a *V* shape configuration is created in the back.

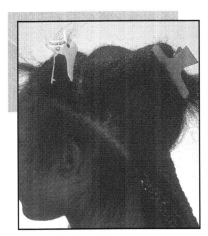

Front to back partings

6. Partings should appear from front to back. Partings in front are curved and continue the diamond shape.

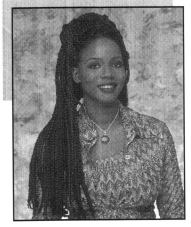

Finished style

7. Braid the hair from scalp to ends, using an underhand, or inverted, technique. Each time you pass a side strand under the center strand, bring the center strand over tightly, so that the side strand becomes the new center strand. Then pass the alternate-side strand under this one.

8. When you reach the ends, pull out a long, small section of hair, wrap it around the braid, knot it, and repeat wrapping and knotting. This holds the tight braid in place and allows it to curve. Then continue to the next parting and repeat the entire procedure. Move up on the head, taking partings according to the pre-planned design.

9. When the entire head is completed, you can heat-seal the ends.

Braid Tapering

The beauty of the casama braid is that the braid is full and wide at the base and tapered off at the ends. The tapered ends usually have a slight curve. To create this effect, the extension material must be shed before it is applied to the head.

1. Hold the required amount of extension material with both hands, about 6 to 10" apart.

2. Slowly pull the hair extension until it becomes uneven at the ends. By being staggered at the ends, the extension material loses its blunt edges.

3. When staggering extension material, or redistributing it in an uneven manner, be aware of the length and size of the braid.

Cornrows and Senegalese Twist (Combo)

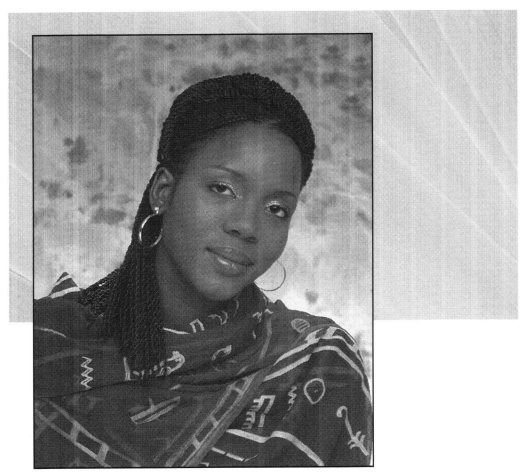

Finished style

This classic combination of micro cornrows and small Senegalese twists was sculpted by Avion Julien of Tulani's Regal Movement of New York.

PART 1

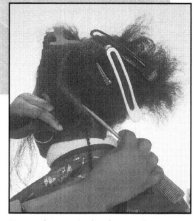

Senegalese twist back—45-degree angle

1. Start in the back by making a diagonal 45-degree angle section to just above the ear. Part off a subsection by making a smaller vertical part to the bottom of the neck.

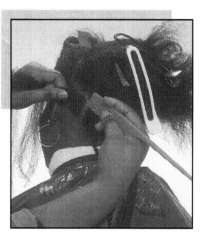

Diagonal parting

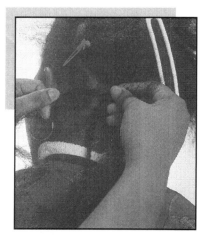

Two equal partings

2. Divide the subsection into 2 equal parts.

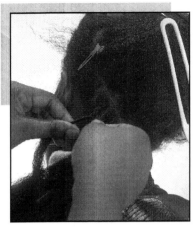

Hold and twist.

3. Make a double twist motion—roll hair strands counterclockwise.

4. Once the extension is twisted close to the scalp, cross over the 2 twisted strands. The role-overlap-roll sequence must be repeated for the entire twist. Tension must be consistent so that the twist remains straight.

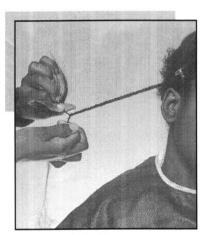

Create a tight braid.

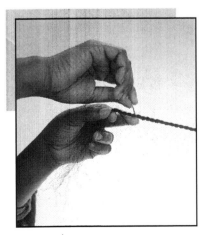

Loop to close.

5. To close, loop ends by separating small numbers of strands and wrapping them around the braid. Singe ends to secure and seal at the desired length.

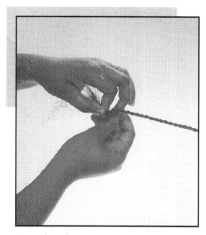

Complete loop.

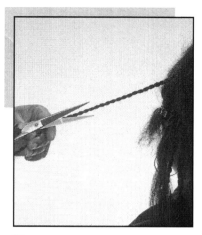

Trim.

6. Trim frizzies, or split ends, from the twist to complete finished style.

PART 2

1. Start at the hairline by parting off the base in the desired size. Vertical parts should be about 1/4" wide.

2. Divide the base into 3 equal portions. Take a pre-measured strip of extension proportionately less than the size of the base. Using the feed-in method, apply small units of extension (10 to 20 hairs) to the hairline.

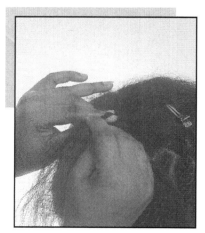

3. Begin the cornrow method. Each time you cross a strand from the outside to the inside center strand, pick up natural hair from the base and add it to the new center strand.

Pick up hair from the base and add to strand.

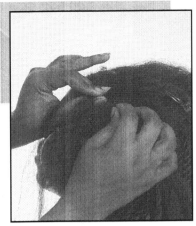

4. With your middle finger, hold the revolution in place. A second strip of extension can be added to the left outside strand.

Hold the revolution in place.

5. After the cornrow base is completed, start the Senegalese twist motion by separating the center strand and adding it to the outside pieces, creating 2 equal portions.

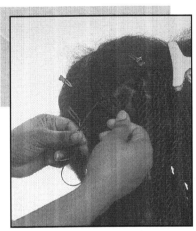

Create 2 equal portions.

6. Continue by starting the double twist motion in order to create the Senegalese twist.

7. Continue until you reach the end. Loop to close; trim and singe ends.

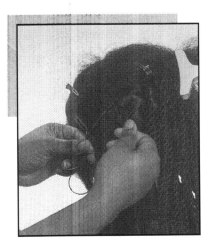

Roll and twist.

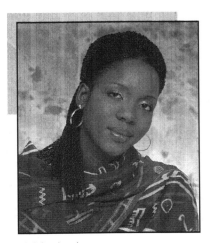

Finished style

INDIVIDUAL BRAIDS

Individual braids may also be known as single or box braids. These are the most versatile to wear, and they are directional—able to move or be swept into updos.

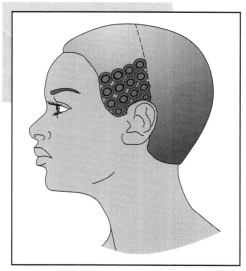

Twist or single braids placement

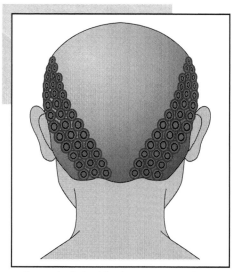

Twist or single braids placement—parting, sectioning, units

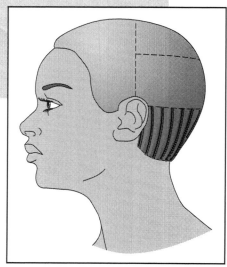

Cornrow—sectioning, parting

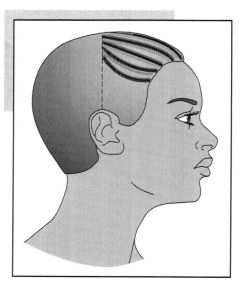

Cornrow placement—parting, sectioning

Whether you use human or synthetic extension or yarn, the variations of the braid are unlimited. Individual braids are traditional and classic. They are as fundamental as cornrows. Skill and practice are necessary in order to master this technique. The individual braid is a 3-strand braid that, if done improperly, can create excessive tension and lead to breakage.

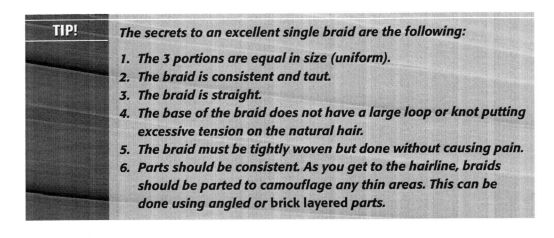

TIP! *The secrets to an excellent single braid are the following:*

1. *The 3 portions are equal in size (uniform).*
2. *The braid is consistent and taut.*
3. *The braid is straight.*
4. *The base of the braid does not have a large loop or knot putting excessive tension on the natural hair.*
5. *The braid must be tightly woven but done without causing pain.*
6. *Parts should be consistent. As you get to the hairline, braids should be parted to camouflage any thin areas. This can be done using angled or brick layered parts.*

Individual Braid

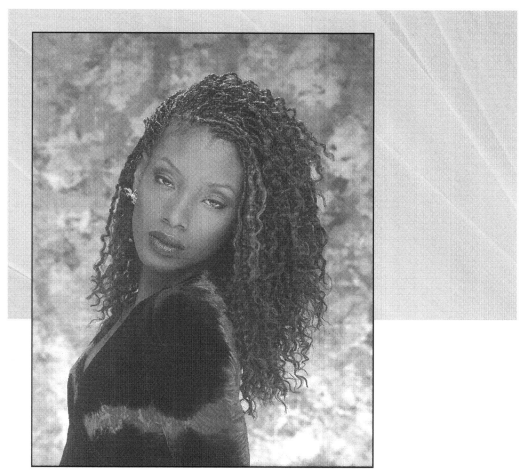

Finished style (shown with Diva Crimp enhancement)

Braid stylist Susan Bishop of Jaha Studio in Silver Springs, Maryland, uses this technique for the individual braid style.

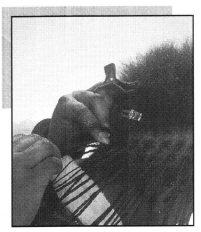

Three equal portions

1. Part the hair in half from ear to ear.

2. With diagonal partings from behind the ear to the nape of the neck, create a subsection with a vertical part for the base size of the braid. Take a pre-determined amount of human hair to begin the braid.

3. Within that subsection, separate the hair into 3 equal parts.

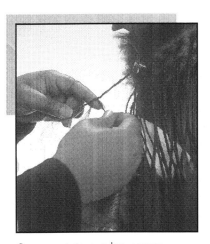

Secure, rotate, overlap, secure.

4. The braid revolution must include the person's natural hair. Each braid is created with the 3-strand braid technique in which the strand on the side is always passed under the center strand.

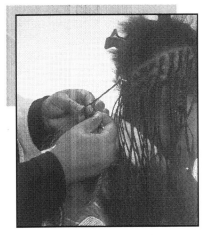

Braid the extension to 2" past the person's natural length for fullness.

5. Continue the braiding sequence with the outer strand crossing under to become the new center strand. Braid the human hair extension to about 2" past the person's natural length. This helps to create fullness.

6. Trim the braid shaft for a finished look.

Diva Crimps

The addition of the crimped texture to braids is an enhancement that has become very popular. It creates dimension and fullness without bulk. It helps to soften the braided style. Many people prefer this look because it gives the braids a loose, directional hair effect.

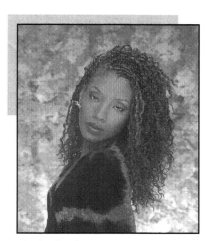

Finished style

1. After the human hair extension is braided and the entire head is complete with braids, lightly spray mist along the whole length of the braid with a diluted setting mixture.
2. Saturate the braid so that its entire depth is covered. It should not be dripping wet, however, because that will increase the drying time.
3. Rebraid the braids. Take about 6 braids, divide them into 3 sets (about 2 braids per section), and braid from the base to the very end. Roll this rebraided hair onto a roller, using a pink or blue (small) perm rod.
4. Allow to dry thoroughly (about 1 hour under a hair dryer).
5. Unbraid the braided strands. Be careful not to disturb the braided extension.
6. Use fingers to take out the double braid. (Flip rebraided hair on the underside and proceed to unravel the braids with an underhand braiding motion.)
7. Trim and shape any uneven ends. The single braids should appear curly and texturized.

Pixie Braids

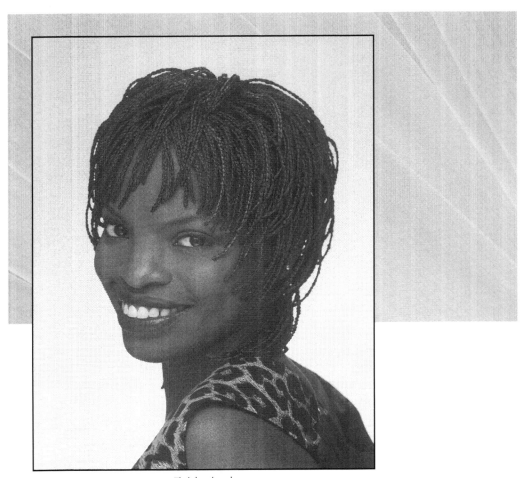

Finished style

The pixie braid style offers a youthful, short braid look. The individual braids are usually small to medium in size. The braids are layered to various lengths, usually framing the face. It is best to use a Kanekalon synthetic hair because this fiber singes better when you are molding the tips. The ends are cut and singed closed for the desired length.

The pixie braid must be tight. This will create a curved braid. There should be a light, airy feel to the braids. The layers create the feathered look when you singe the tips wherever necessary to complete the style. Always be aware of the natural hair length so that you do not burn the hair. The hair must be short for this technique, and the finished braid can be slightly longer than the natural length. Singe the braid to be 1 to 2" longer than the natural hair.

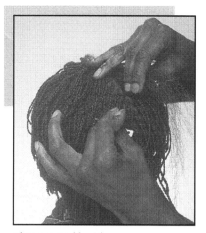

Three-strand braid sequence

1. Follow steps of individual braid instruction to start pixie braids.

2. Maintain the 3-strand, outside-to-inside strand underhand braiding technique. Keep the braid stitch close.

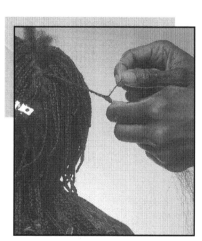

First loop

3. To hold the tight stitch taut, double loop the ends. Bring together the 3 strands; hold in one hand. With the other hand, separate several strands out from the braid, loop over and around, and pull through the loop. Repeat.

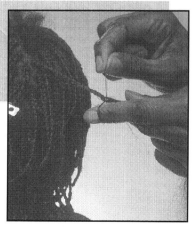

Second loop

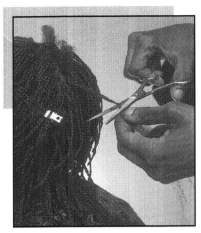

Trim.

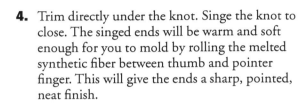

4. Trim directly under the knot. Singe the knot to close. The singed ends will be warm and soft enough for you to mold by rolling the melted synthetic fiber between thumb and pointer finger. This will give the ends a sharp, pointed, neat finish.

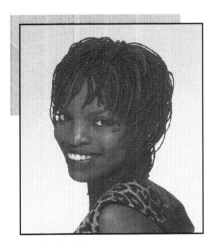

Finished style

Flat Twists

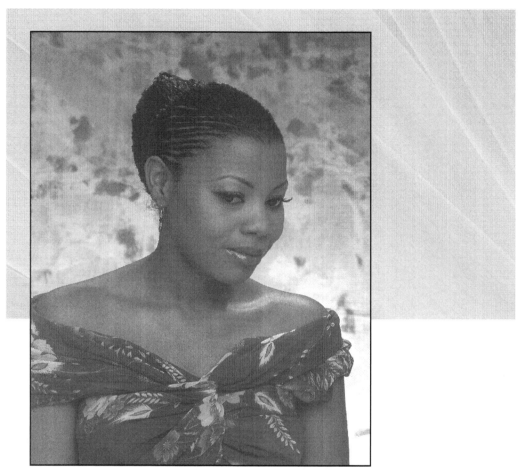

Finished style

Flat twists are a great alternative for people with medium- to shoulder-length hair. These twists are regal, soft, and easily sculpted into a day or evening look. Flat twists are a wonderful option for women who are interested in wearing their hair natural, but who do not want extensions or a woven braided look. Whether the hair is relaxed or chemical-free, this sculpted style offers an elegant and sophisticated crown of glory.

The flat twist is a 2-strand, flat-on-the-scalp braid. The pattern resembles the flat spiral on a candy cane. Master braider Cecelia Hinds of Uzuri Braids in Washington, D.C., uses this technique. You twist 2 strands of equal proportions onto the scalp, picking up natural hair with every revolution. Most flat twist styles can last for 2 to 3 weeks.

To maintain this style, no shampooing is required. Cover the hair nightly with a satin scarf. Oil the scalp as needed.

"Lin Twist"—Flat Twist with Lin

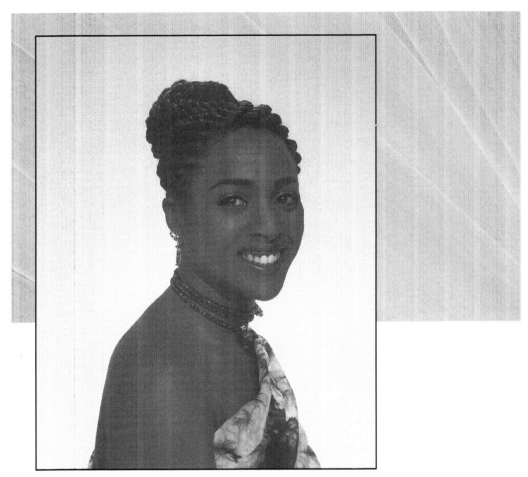

Finished style

Lin twists are the new classic of updo braiding styles. They give medium- to shoulder-length hair dimension and diversity. The style can last 3 to 4 weeks. It can be done in 2 hours and is a quick alternative for people who want extensions incorporated into their braid style. This technique also has been mastered by Cecelia Hinds of Uzuri Braids.

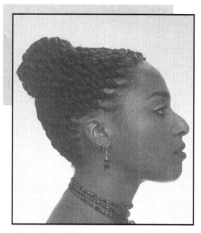

Lin twist—side

1. The 2-strand twist can be performed using the roll-and-twist method at the hairline. Place the lin flat on top of the 2 equal portions. Secure the lin to each base with the double twist sequence, picking up natural hair with each revolution.

2. Pre-plan the style so that it fits the contour of the head along the sides and back.

3. Gather the extended ends into a French roll or inverted cornrow; pin and tuck.

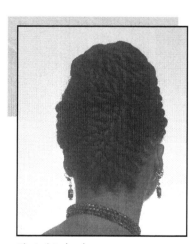

Lin twist—back

The African Kurl—Twist Out

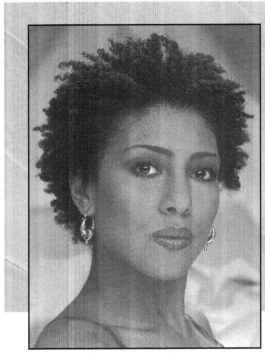
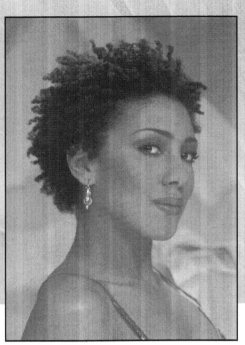

Finished style   African kurl—side

The African kurl is a versatile style that is easy to care for. The textured tresses can be worn at the office or for an evening out. This style softly flows and bounces to all the urban beats.

1. The hair is double twisted on the individual braid pattern. This is a double twist set—the hair is wet and sprayed with a setting lotion.

2. After the hair is totally dry, this twist style can be worn for 2 or 3 weeks. Oil the scalp sparingly once or twice a week.

3. After a week or two, if you want to change the style, you can un-twist the twists. We call it "twist out." The twist out can be done on the same day as the set for a beautiful, fresh look. Some people opt to wait 1 to 2 weeks before opening the twist in order to add versatility and long life to the crimped tresses.

4. Separate each twist for a full, bountiful look. Avoid disturbing the wave pattern. Use fingers to fan out the twist. A small pick can be used to remove parts and to lift. Only use a pick at the base of the scalp. The resulting style will last 2 to 3 weeks. Use moisturizing sheen when necessary.

5. This set can also be applied to relaxed, straight hair. Drying time is 1 hour, and perm rods can be used for a fuller, spiral effect.

African Kurl and Flat Twist "Sunburst"

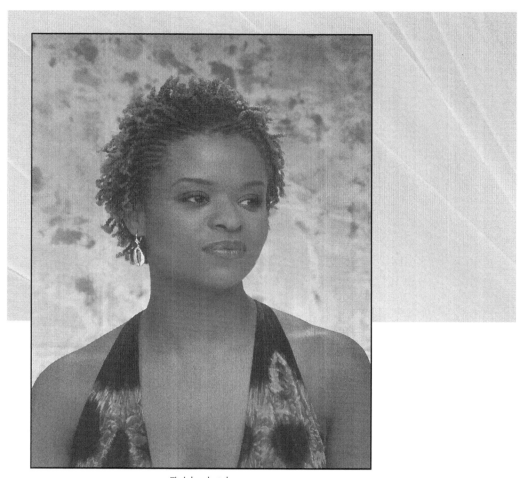

Finished style

This combination of natural twists is fresh and youthful. The styles mix a curly look with the sculpted flat twist, which spreads sunshine to every face. The tighter the coil pattern, the more texture the curls will have. These curls are versatile and can last for up to 6 weeks.

For more fullness you can do a twist out. You can un-twist both the curls and the flat twist for styling options.

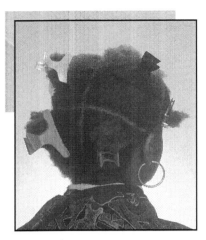

Four sections

1. Shampoo and deep condition the hair. Towel dry, squeezing out excess moisture. Hair should be damp but not dripping wet.

2. With tail comb, divide the hair in half from ear to ear. Then divide the back portion of the hair into 4 sections.

3. Beginning at the nape, lightly apply a pinch of water-soluble gel to each subsection. With a horizontal parting, sub-divide vertically into 1/4" partings. Overlap equal portions while moving counterclockwise and do a 2-strand twist to the ends of the strand. The twist must be tight, so revolutions should be close together to form the curl pattern.

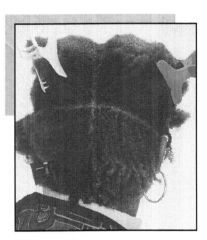

Close together to form curl

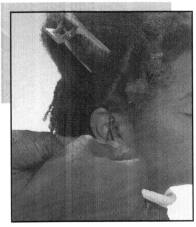

Lower side, 2 strands

4. When the back is completed, move to the side and repeat the twist movement.

5. Dampen hair in front with a spray bottle of water and oil to keep moist. Flat twist damp hair into a small, sculpted pattern. Place person under dryer until hair is completely dry.

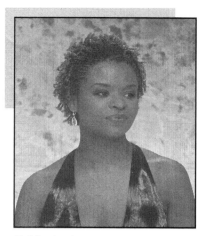

Finished style

6. Lightly oil scalp and finish with moisturizing spray sheen.

LOCKS

Nubian Coils

Styling the hair in Nubian coils is the first step toward locking hair. Nubian coils are small spiral curls, usually short to medium in length. The texture of the hair determines the formation, or coil pattern. Some coil patterns are tighter, or closer together, than others. If the coil pattern is smaller, then the coil will be tight. The reverse also holds true: the larger the wave or curl formation, the larger in size the actual coil will be. By examining the coil pattern of several strands of hair over the entire head, you will be able to determine the size and characteristics of the coil formation.

Examine the hair to determine the coil pattern. Check 3 different areas of the head:

1. The nape (the "kitchen") is usually tight; very coily or curly; and dense.

2. The side hairline is usually slightly less coily or curly and may be thinner. Look for damage or alopecia.

3. The crown may have the least curl or wave pattern. For some menopausal women, this area may thin or bald. However, this area is usually rich with a dense concentration of hair.

The average person has several textures of hair, from grey wiry to fine coily. What this means is that you must be aware of the differences and apply the necessary techniques based on the hair texture to get the best results before locking.

Nubian coils are the "pre-lock phase" before African locks, or dread locks, as they are often called. This pre-locked phase is a beautiful style in itself and can be worn to work or for play. It is neat yet at the same time loose in structure. When done initially, Nubian coils are flat and contoured to the head. When you use different styling gels, a shiny/glossy glow gives the coils their finished look. However, after about 48 hours, the coil "puffs" open slightly—just enough to expand the spiral and soften the curl. The coil formation is still in place and can last for up to 6 weeks. The life of this coiled style depends on the size of the coil. Smaller coils last longer, and the tighter the coil or curl pattern, the longer the style will last, since this style is the preparatory style for African locks.

It is necessary to know whether the person intends to lock or just wants to wear his or her hair in a natural coiled style. The person who is interested in locking is at a higher commitment level, physically, emotionally, and spiritually willing to invest the time—which is usually 6 months to a year—for the locks to solidify and mature.

Hair locking is a natural coiling process of textured curly hair that happens without the use of combs or chemicals. The hair meshes and spirals within itself, interlocking and adhering until the joined strands become a tight, dense unit, or lock. The hair locks in slow developmental stages, which can take anywhere from 6 months to a year depending on the length, density, and coil pattern. Cultivating locks is a process, a journey into self-discovery and acceptance of genetic and cultural inheritance.

There are several ways to cultivate locks, such as double twisting, wrapping with cord or wire, braiding with or without extension, or simply not disturbing the hair by not combing or brushing the lock (as the Rastafarians of Jamaica do); if the hair is just left to its own natural course, it will lock. However, it will not have a groomed, manicured look. I refer to this type of locks as "organic" locks. Cultivated African locks have symmetry. The goal to grooming locks is to create uniform tresses that will turn heads when the person is well groomed. Symmetry is not easy to achieve with textured hair. Although the hair is programmed genetically to coil, no two coils are exactly alike. It is your responsibility to develop a system that promotes symmetry in the textured hair. Three basic methods of locking are (1) comb, (2) palm roll, and (3) braid or extension.

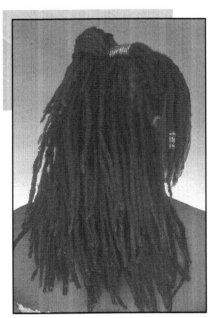

Mature locks

The most effective techniques that use the natural coil pattern are the comb technique and the palm roll method. The comb technique can be most effective during the early stages of locking, while the coil is still open. This method of coiling entails placing the comb at the base of the coil and, in a rotating motion, spiraling the hair into a curl. With each revolution the comb moves down until it reaches the end of the hair shaft. This method offers a great tight coil and is excellent on short (1 to 3") hair.

The second method of grooming and starting locks is the palm roll method. This method is the gentlest on the hair and guides it through all the natural stages of locking. Palm rolling takes advantage of the hair's natural ability to coil. The following description shows how to use the palm roll method to create a coiled style.

Nubian Coils—Pre-locking Phase

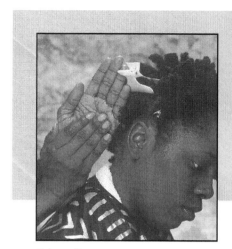

Palm rolling

1. To begin, shampoo and condition the hair. Then towel blot the hair, squeezing out excess moisture so that the hair is damp but not wet.

2. Next, part the hair in horizontal rows from the nape all the way to the front hairline. Then divide the first horizontal row at the nape into equal size subsections. The subsections can be square, circular, triangular, or rectangular; the size of the individual sections and their shape depend on the desired finished look. Before palm rolling, use hair clips to hold the hair around the subsection out of the way.

3. Beginning at the nape on the far side, take the hair within the first subsection and lightly apply a pinch of gel, using your right forefinger and thumb. Then pinch the hair near the scalp and twist it 1 full counterclockwise revolution. (If you are left-handed, use your left hand to pinch the hair, but always turn it counterclockwise.)

4. With one smooth motion, pass the hair from your right hand to your left hand, tuck the hair into the recession near the thumb, and fold your thumb down to hold the hair in place. Position your left hand behind your right hand so that the left fingertips are at the right wrist. Slide your right hand back while sliding the left hand forward.

5. When the hair is between your palms, pull out your thumb so that the hair is rolled between your palms. When the fingertips of your right hand are near the left-hand wrist, fold your thumb back down to recapture the hair.

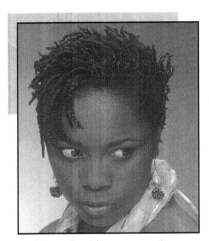

Nubian coils with yarn extension

6. So that the hair is always rolled in a counterclockwise direction, reposition the left hand behind the right hand and repeat the palm rolling technique. Each time you roll the hair, move progressively down the hair shaft. When you reach the ends, place the lock down neatly and begin again with the adjacent subsection.

7. When each subsection in the first horizontal row has been completed, move up to the next horizontal row and sub-divide it as before. If you rolled the previous subsections from right to left, this time work from left to right. Continue this pattern all the way to the crown. As you work up the head, include the side sections. Always maintain a degree of moisture by using the spray bottle as needed. Also, apply the same amount of gel to each subsection.

8. When you reach the crown, continue palm rolling subsections, directing them to move toward the back. When you reach the top of the head, move around the person to accommodate the desired finished style. If the person wants the front individualized, for instance, if a few sections are to move onto the forehead, reposition yourself in front of the person to palm roll these subsections.

9. When all the hair has been palm rolled, place the person under a hood dryer set on low heat. Dry the hair completely, but no more than necessary.

10. When the hair is completely dry, finish the style by applying a light oil to add sheen.

11. Single braids with yarn are a lock alternative which is added to the front to frame the face. The ends are looped and singed to the desired length.

African Locks

The ultimate in natural hair care is the textured richness of hair locking. Throughout the continent of Africa, various tribes have practiced this art form and cultural expression of beauty enhancement. The people of the Pokot, Massai, Mau Mau, Kau, Ashanti, and Fulani tribes, as well as many others, practice some form of locking. Some tribes use mud or a red clay with straw or hay to perform the grooming technique.

Locks are what the Afro was in the 1960s: a symbol of freedom, cultural empowerment, and identity, as well as a seed to self-acceptance. Ona Osirio-Maat, a locktician for 11 years, is the creator of the *LockSmyth method,* a lock technique that incorporates a special, rhythmical palm rolling technique. Osirio-Maat stated during a phone interview with the author, "Locked hair is the ultimate natural hair statement. It says you have come home . . . finally. The self-love and appreciation that has been gained from 'growing' through the process can have tremendous transformative power surrounding the 'locker' life. People usually undergo some deeper level of self-evaluation as they return for professional cultivation of their locks, and the stories center around their hair getting longer and stronger. Also, there are stories about the strength their locks silently display. As a locktician, I witness the internal growth of my clients as well as the inches of hair flowing down their backs. Their pride is tempered by the humility of the process. Instead of running fast, hard, and long distances from the kink, they changed their perspective and began to embrace the coil."

The Developmental Stages of Hair Locking

Depending on the coil pattern, density, and length of hair, the locking process may vary from 6 to 12 months to lock the entire head.

Phase I Pre-lock Stage—Hair is soft and is coiled into spiral configurations. The coil is smooth and the end is open. The coil has a shiny, or a glossy, texture.

Phase II Sprouting Stage—Hair begins to interlace and mesh. The separate units begin to "puff up" and expand. The units are no longer glossy, thin, and smooth. Little bulbs, or knots, form at the middle or ends of the coiled unit, indicating that the coil is starting to close. This "plumping" of the lock may give the head an unkempt look. Avoid over-grooming or excessive twisting at this phase. The length starts to shrink because the coil is solidifying. This "frizzy" look is part of the process. Here is where patience and desire are virtues—and the person's level of commitment is tested. This is also the stage in which some sections of the head will be totally locked, while other portions of the head will still have soft and open coils. Be aware of the different coil patterns and the density of the hair in each area.

Phase III Growing Stage—The hair strands adhere to one another, creating a network of tresses within each coiled unit. You can feel interlacing and meshing by squeezing the lock. You can feel a bulb at the end of each lock. The locking process starts at the middle or ends of the unit, not at the scalp. Hair begins to regain length. The lock still may be frizzy, yet solid in some areas. Locks are closed at the ends, dense, and dull, not reflecting light to get any sheen.

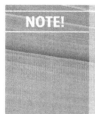 **NOTE!** *Textured curly, coily hair does not reflect light the way straight hair does. The person may complain about the dullness, or the lack of luster. Again, this is part of the process. Reassure the person that this perceived dullness is what creates the lock. One can add oils, which allow the light to reflect off the oils and give the hair a gloss.*

Phase IV Maturation Stage—The lock is now totally closed at the end. The unit is interlaced and meshed, giving the hair a tighter, rope-like look, except where there is new growth at the base. The network of intertwined strands is tight and hard to the touch. The hair grows at a rapid rate. Whether the strands are in the *anagen cycle* or *telogen cycle* of growth, all the hair is fused together; because the hair is not combed or brushed, there is little shedding. The hair stays within the locked unit. New sprouts spring up between mature locks. In some cases, the hair forms whole new locks.

 NOTE! *Some textures will not close at the end. A single curl or wave may exist at the end of the lock, giving the lock the appearance of being open. The maturation stage will still continue.*

Phase V Atrophy Stage—After several years of maturation (the usual time varies between 7 and 10 years), the lock may start to weaken, or atrophy, at the ends. The smaller the lock, the more fragile it is, and the more likely it is that the atrophy will occur. The larger the lock, the more durable it is, and the degeneration may never occur. This atrophy stage usually occurs at the nape of the neck and around the frontal and peripheral hairlines. When the person's hair starts to weaken, consult with him or her and make sure it is part of a natural locking process and not due to physical or emotional stress. Here is how to tell the difference:

1. Thinning and breakage at the ends are signs of a degenerative process and part of the locks' life cycle; excessive dryness can accelerate this process.

2. Thinning and breakage at the base, or scalp, are the body's warning signals that something is internally or externally imbalanced.

How to Cultivate and Groom Locks

There is an effective 7-step procedure for grooming and cultivating locks:

1. To start locks, use the palm roll technique described earlier in the chapter.

2. Avoid over-twisting. With each revolution, move down the shaft to avoid over-spiraling the hair.

3. During the first 3 months, the person should have the locks groomed every 3 or 4 weeks.

4. Grooming may entail the following:

- Herbal shampoo.

- Hot oil treatment.

- Herbal rinse or acid rinse.

- Re-rolling, cultivating, or manicuring.

- Trim (optional).

- Styling (texturizing, to include crimping, curling, braiding, and so on).

- Watering: Spritzing with water helps keep locks or natural curls clean. The weight of water helps the lock drop down in length and brings lint to the surface. Keeping the hair wet is one of the keys to lock growth and promotes the natural curling of hair.

5. Always remove lock debris, lint, and excess oils embedded in locks.

6. Avoid using heavy petroleum or waxy oils. Use diluted moisturizing and water-soluble gels when rolling the hair.

7. Once the locks are fully matured, the hair can be shampooed more often.

 CAUTION! *Be careful not to dry out the hair. Use lemon rinses and acid rinses to loosen the lock debris after each shampoo for deep cleansing. Follow with light hot oil treatments to the scalp.*

Locked hair may appear dull when not properly cared for. Locks do, however, have a beautiful sheen when healthy and clean. The sheen is subtly understated and soft because, like most natural fibers, locks have a matte finish; this finish is a part of their natural beauty and uniqueness. Avoid applying large amounts of braid oil or moisturizing sheen to create more shine; this contributes to lock sediment build-up. Once or twice a week, small amounts of natural oil (dime size) can be applied to the scalp and massaged through the hair to create luster. With locks, "less is more."

Styling and Texturizing Locks

At the salon Tendrils in Brooklyn, New York, texture is used to enhance the natural tress. The finer the lock, the more versatility the stylist will have to create new looks. To eliminate breakage, avoid putting too much stress on the hair. Remember: Thin locks are fragile.

- Texturizing—On damp locks, lightly spray a setting lotion. Braid or twist the entire length. Add a perm rod or clip to hold the end. The hair must be completely dry before unbraiding or twisting out in order to get style.

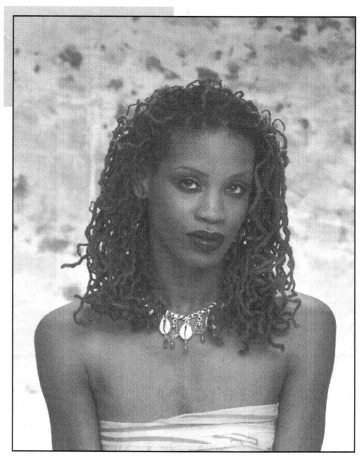

Finished style

■ Tendrils/Spirals—On damp locks, lightly spray a setting lotion to cover the entire lock surface. Take a perm rod (pink, purple, or white) and vertically wind the lock around the rod, starting at the end of the hair and moving up toward the scalp.

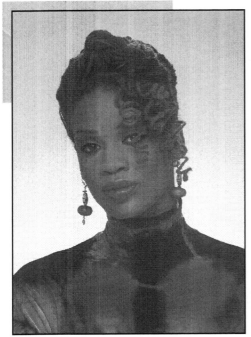

Upswept locks—spiral curl

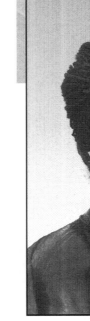

Upswept locks—side

■ Updo Sweeps—Roll, twist, braid, pin, and tuck. Create chignons, buns, French rolls, and inverted braids—be as creative as your hair will let you. There are no limits!

MATERIALS FOR EXTENSIONS

There are a variety of materials that are available for the purpose of extending textured hair. The life of the style, however, will always be determined by the materials used. As braid extensions become more popular, more varieties of quality and price will be available. Though it may save money to buy the least expensive product, beware that you may not get the desired results. In other words, the extension material is critical to the final outcome of your hair design.

When buying a new product, buy in small quantities and test the fiber on a small section of hair before using it on the whole head.

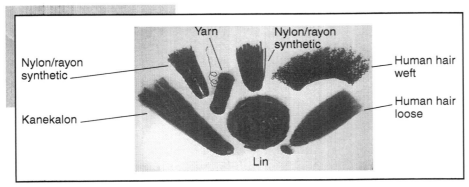

Extension materials

The following list may help you to decide what extension material to use:

1. Kanekalon—It is a synthetic fiber of excellent quality. It is designed to have a texture similar to that of African hair types. It does not reflect light, which means it has less shine. It is durable and holds up to shampooing and styling. When being used in braiding the hair, it is smooth to the scalp and fingers, which is very important because it means it does not cut or damage natural hair as other, less expensive products do. It generally has a softer feel and tangles less than other synthetics. It comes in a variety of colors. It is versatile and easy to match with natural hair colors. Kanekalon costs more than most synthetics but is of a better quality—not only according to manufacturers, but also according to many braid stylists. This extension material finishes well when you are using the singeing method; it burns safely and seals quickly.

2. Nylon/Rayon Synthetic—This product is less expensive and readily available. The quality can vary depending on the brand name. You must be familiar with the brands in order to get a decent quality. In general, the less expensive synthetic hair tangles more and can damage natural hair. Nylon and rayon have been known to cut or break the hair. They are often less durable after repeated shampooing. They also reflect light and leave hair very shiny. Stylists must be cautious when choosing the quality of the extension material. Nylon and rayon synthetics, however, come in more varieties of color than Kanekalon. However, these materials do not burn well when you are using the singe method to close synthetic extensions. The warm plastic melts too quickly, holds heat, and can burn and blister the skin.

NOTE! *It has been my experience that when the hair is shampooed regularly, the natural hair begins to expand—but the Kanekalon or other synthetic hair does not. As the natural hair expands, the tension at the base of the braid with the extension increases.*

CAUTION! *Warning: This extension material finishes poorly when you are using the singeing method; melted fibers can stick to the skin and burn. Avoid this material when singeing.*

3. Human Hair—This material is the most confusing of the fibers and is somewhat mysterious. Most of the product is imported from Asia. It is a closed market, and very little is known about how the supposed human hair is produced or processed. Some of it is imported from Europe, and small amounts are from Africa. Although the label may say "human hair," buyer beware—all that glitters is not gold. The buyer must select hair from a reputable dealer or wholesaler of this product to be assured of its quality. Pre-packaged human hair is generally less expensive than that which is customized by a wholesaler. If a wholesaler is not available in your area, consider mail order.

This material (supposedly) is derived from human hair and is processed into hundreds of colors and textures. It is versatile, soft, and tangle-free. Although the material is extremely expensive, sometimes overpriced, it moves and feels like natural hair. It expands along with human hair when it is washed, which may also change the desired results and the life of a particular hairstyle. It can easily slip from the base of the braid. But unlike Kanekalon, it can be reused, if properly cleaned and combed. This product is ideal for those who are allergic to the synthetic products. To finish braid styles with human hair you can use thermal curling tools and set the hair for crimps.

4. Human Hair Weft—Wefted human hair has all the advantages of loose human hair, except that when it is shampooed it does not expand to the point that it can slip from the base. The material is sewn together on a woven strip that interlaces with the individual human hair strands. Wefted human hair is a great alternative to add dimension, length, and color to a person's natural hair. Wefted hair is sewn with a needle and thread into a braided cornrow track and netting.

5. Yarn—Traditional yarn material is used to make fabric for sweaters, hats, and so on. But now it is being used to adorn textured African hair. When braided or wrapped, it is light and soft and detangles easily. Yarn comes in many colors. The most commonly used is black or brown for a more natural look. Yarn is different than synthetic fibers because it does not reflect any light. It is not glossy. It gives the braid style a matte finish and can give braids a "locked" look. But be careful when choosing yarns. Some black yarns have a blue or green tint. A yarn may appear jet black in the store but, in the light, reflect green. Always hold yarn to the light before purchasing. Yarn is very inexpensive and easy to find. Also, the yarn can be cotton or a nylon blend, and though it may expand when shampooed, it does not slip from the base. So, braid styles that use yarns are durable. Do not burn yarns if they are 100% cotton. Finish braids with a neat knot.

6. Lin—This is a beautiful wool fiber made in France and imported from Africa. Like yarn, it has a matte finish and gives off little shine. It only comes in black and brown. Lin can be purchased in packages of 25 m or 24 yds. It comes on a roll and is used in any length and size. Often used for Senegalese twists and "corkscrew" styles, this fiber cannot be singed. It is cottony and very flammable. Braid styles using lin are generally not shampooed often.

7. Yak—This strong textured fiber comes from the domestic ox, usually found in the mountains of Tibet and central Asia. The hairs on the ox are long on the sides and the back. These hairs are shaven and processed to be used alone or blended with human hair. The variety of blends usually creates a more African texture when yak is used in wigs. Small mixtures of yak with human hair help to remove the manufactured shine.

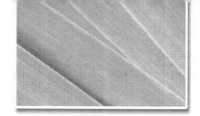

Index

9912174R0

Made in the USA
Lexington, KY
09 June 2011